the Second Mile

MORE REFLECTIONS from the AUTHOR of
A RUNNING COMMENTARY

ROGER PRESCOTT

THE SECOND MILE

5823/ISBN 0-89536-739-4

With thanks for their

unconditional encouragement

this book is dedicated to . . .

Gerald R. Prescott

and

Elsie M. Prescott,

my father and mother

CONTENTS

Acknowledgments 8

Preface 11

How to Get the Most From This Book 13

The Flat Tire 15

Fat Can't Catch Hold If You Keep Movin' 16

Ruthville 17

High Tech / High Touch 18

Making a List 19

What a Racket! 20

It's Great to Be Alive 22

Bending and Whirling 24

A Child Again 25

The Pig's Advantage 27

The Best Things in Life Are Free 28

Live For the Moment 30

The Young Nurse 31

Watching It Get Dark 32

Prejudiced in Your Favor 33

A Bridge of Instant Rapport 35

Overcoming "Din City" 36

Fargo Is Asleep 38

A '49 Ford 39

Festina Lente 41

The Wood Pile 42

My Daily Run 43

No Time to Be in a Hurry 44

Runners and Pilots 45

Our Thoughts Are Handed to Us 46

Words of Cheer 47

A Cold Morning 48

Poetry 49

Hello 51

A Fragile Prize 52

All Those T-Shirts 53

The Lost Datebook 54

Middle Age Forgetfulness 55

Nothing Is Really Frightening 57

Only Three Things Ever Scared Me 58

Birds 59

Puddles 60

The Unfair Distribution of Suffering 61

Two Can 62

Days Away 63

The Great Leveler 64

An Announcement of Reality 65

Older Runners 66

Feelings 67

Inspired to Run 68

After Everything Was Supposed to Be Over 69

Guaranteed Hierarchical Privileges 70

Self Esteem 71

A Great Time Was Had By All 72

A Happy Gasp. 73

A Sort of a Prayer 74

Sentences That Sing 75

Fixed, Sure, and Regular. 77

Let Me Be What I Can Be 78

Compulsion 80

You Don't Have to Sit on That Bench 81

In Between Funerals 82

Church Choirs 84

Names 85

The Importance of Friends. 86

Sex Is a Hot Item 87

Curing Ourselves 89

Be a Friend to Yourself 90

A Minor Rebirth 91

Free Space. 92

The Poet and the Runner 93

After Suicide 95

Cats Are Always on the Wrong Side of Doors 96

Don't Judge a Runner's Happiness By the Width of the Grin   97

Don't Sweat the Small Stuff 98

We Buried Mom Today. 99

Family Memories 101

Speed Work. 102

Cars We Have Known. 103

ACKNOWLEDGMENTS

Grateful acknowledgment is made to the following publishers and authors:

After Suicide, by John H. Hewett, The Westminster Press, copyright 1980.

The Art of Teaching, by Gilbert Highet, Random House — Alfred A. Knopf — Vintage Books, copyright 1957. Used by permission.

The Battle of Faith, by Edward Sidney Kiek, James Clarke, London, copyright 1938.

Beginner's Running Guide, by Hal Higdon, World Publications, P.O. Box 366, Mountain View, California, copyright 1978. Used by permission.

Blessed Is the Ordinary, by Gerhard E. Frost. Copyright 1980, Gerhard E. Frost. Published by Winston Press, Inc., 430 Oak Grove, Minneapolis, Minnesota 55403. All rights reserved. Used by permission.

The Book of Comfort, by Alvin N. Rogness, Augsburg Publishing House, copyright 1979. Used by permission.

The Complete Book of Running, by James F. Fixx, Random House, copyright 1977. Used by permission.

The Deserted Rooster, by Ric Masten, Sunflower Ink, Palo Colorado Road, Carmel, California 93923. Copyright 1982. Used by permission of the author.

Eighth Day of Creation, by Elizabeth O'Connor, copyright 1971; used by permission of Word Books, publisher, Waco, Texas 76796.

Embodiment, by James B. Nelson, Augsburg Publishing House. Copyright 1978. Reprinted by permission.

The Genesee Diary, by Henri J. M. Nouwen, Doubleday, copyright 1976, by Henri J. M. Nouwen. Reprinted by permission of Doubleday and Company, Inc.

Growth Counseling, by Howard Clinebell, Abingdon Press, copyright 1979. Used by permission.

Healing and Wholeness, by John A. Sanford, Paulist Press, copyright 1977. Used by permission.

How to Be Your Own Best Friend, by Mildred Newman and Bernard Berkowitz with Jean Owen, Random House, copyright 1971. Used by permission.

"The Incredible World of Cats" from *Yankee* Magazine, October, 1980. Used with permission.

PREFACE

Somewhere recently I read the words, "God hides things by putting them near us." So maybe if we are able to do our usual things in an unusual way (like paying extra attention), we might find a new awareness of the presence of God in our lives. That's what I've been trying to do during these "middle years" of my life.

The reflections in this little book have grown out of my daily run. For approximately forty-five minutes each morning you can find me loping along a road somewhere, listening to creation around and within, and letting my unconscious mind lift up thoughts from the past. This running starts the juices of the mind. When I'm on the road scenes from earlier days are handed to me by my unconscious. Then parts from my regular reading are brought to mind; and scripture passages too. In these pages some of those pieces are blended together.

The thoughts here are intended to sharpen your eye for the ordinary, and maybe even help you find a measure of peace in your life. I hope, too, it will add a new dimension to your days, keeping you "hope centered" and more keenly aware of God's presence around you. After all, what Karen Horney once said is quite true: "Life itself remains a very effective therapy."

Read one page a day, letting these ideas be springboards for your own reflection and dreaming.

Roger Prescott, Pastor
Lutheran Social Services
of North Dakota
Box 389
Fargo, ND 58107

The figure of a labourer — some furrows in a ploughed field — a bit of sand, sea, and sky — are serious subjects, so difficult, but at the same time so beautiful, that it is indeed worthwhile to devote one's life to the task of expressing the poetry hidden in them.

— Vincent Van Gogh

HOW TO GET THE MOST FROM THIS BOOK

Here are some suggestions for getting maximum benefit from this book:

1. Read, discuss, and experience these readings with people you love and cherish.

2. Take time from your busy schedule to "listen to your life." Do that by reading one-page-a-day and let your mind spin off wherever it will.

3. When a passage of scripture intrigues you, read "around" it as you have time.

4. As you use the book, jot down your own ideas, scripture thoughts, questions or reactions in a small notebook. Let that be a start of your own growth journal.

5. Write to me with your insights, thoughts and readings that have been meaningful to you. I'm always anxious for dialogue with those who are "leaning into life."

Rev. Roger Prescott
Box 389
Fargo, ND 58107
(701) 235-7341

THE FLAT TIRE

Returning from a run, I notice one of my tires is flat. What a drag! It's enough to push a guy into buying a new car. (You know how the mind works). Open the trunk. Get out the gear. Hope the spare is up. Remove hub cap. Now, which way do these nuts turn? Why do some tighten one way and others another? Uhhh! That's not it. Try again. Am I just weak, or is it the wrong way? Frankly, I'd rather be running.

Today I learned a lesson,
the simplest kind of lesson —
from a fruit jar cover!

My first turn was wrong;
but I was stubborn,
and I was strong.

The second was more wrong
because I was strong.

And now it sticks.

How sad to be strong
(and stubborn)
when you're wrong.

> — Gerhard E. Frost
> *Kept Moments*
> (Winston Press, 1982), p. 76

> I do not understand my own actions.
> For I do not do what I want, but I do
> the very thing I hate.
> — Romans 7:15

— Recall something you have done that was just the opposite of what it should have been.

FAT CAN'T CATCH HOLD IF YOU KEEP MOVIN'

Every now and again when I'm caught up in the euphoria of a long run I wonder afresh how I got started with this nourishing addiction. Today I read some words that help me understand again. "Keep movin'," said Satchel Paige, "and the fat will never settle anywhere. Fat can't catch hold if you keep moving." Isn't that superb!? It says a lot to me today. And in some mysterious way it speaks to why I started to run.

Paige worked as a coach for the now defunct Tulsa Oilers in 1976, after a long career in professional baseball. While at Tulsa little leaguers would troop to him nightly for an autograph. He gave each a small white business card and said, "Look on the back. That's where my secret is." The youngsters turned over the card and read old Satchel Paige's Six Rules for a Happy Life:

— *Avoid fried meats which angry up the blood.*

— *If your stomach disputes you, lie down and pacify it with cool thoughts.*

— *Keep the juices flowing by jangling around gently as you move.*

— *Go very light on vices such as carrying on in society. The social ramble ain't restful.*

— *Avoid running at all times.*

— *Don't look back. Something may be gaining on you.*

I wish he hadn't said that about running, but then, I bet he meant "Avoid *hurrying* at all costs." I can live with that!

> Let your moderation be known unto all.
> — Philippians 4:5 (KJV)

Which of these Six Rules of Satchel Paige make the most sense to you today?

RUTHVILLE

I am passing through Ruthville, North Dakota, just north of Minot. I stop to see if they have a Post Office so that I can mail a note to Ruth with the postmark "Ruthville." No such luck. They tell me at the gas station that this place has a Minot address. Rural Route.

I think back to four years ago when Ruth got me started in my addiction. She was home from Gustavus for the summer and wanted me to run with her. We began at the Y. This was a real turning point in my life. Eventually she went back to school . . . and I just kept on running.

Returning to memory also is how thirsty Ruthie was as a baby — all that milk she drank (all night sometimes!) — and I'm suddenly dry. The pop machine spits out a Tab after I drop in 55 cents. My money returns too. Ruthville is a lucky place for me. And lucky for me my daughter started me running. Thanks, Bug!

One of the reasons we experience so much difficulty with our gifts is that parents have thought their chief function in life to be feeding, clothing, and educating the young. However, their really important ministry is to listen to their children and enable them to uncover the special blueprint that is theirs . . . Instead of telling our children what they should do and become, we must be humble before their wisdom . . .
— Elizabeth O'Connor
Eighth Day of Creation
(Word Books, 1971), p. 18

And they went on to another village.
— Luke 9:56

Recall a small town that has a memory for you. What person is associated with it?

HIGH TECH / HIGH TOUCH

I stop running for a moment to pick up a bunch of keys lying on the street. I look all around as I wonder how to return them to a no doubt worried owner. No one is around and it's still dark. I recall how I retrace my steps when I lose something. So, not able to think of anything better, I put them back in the same spot.

Our human family has used keys for a long time now, but when some of us carry around seven or eight (or more) of them, something has changed. Obviously, we have moved toward a society with much more technology.

In his book, *Megatrends*, societal analyst John Naisbitt uses a formula he calls high tech/high touch to describe the way we have responded to technology:

> *"What happens is that whenever new technology is introduced into society, there must be a counterbalancing human response — that is, high touch — or the technology is rejected. The more high tech, the more high touch."*
> — John Naisbitt
> *Megatrends: Ten New Directions Transforming Our Lives.*
> (Warner Books, 1982), p. 39

How I'd like to have done some "high-touch" by returning those keys in person!

> . . . But when he still did not open
> the doors of the roof chamber, they
> took the key and opened them . . .
> — Judges 3:25

What are some examples of "high-tech" living that bothers you these days? To get your mind moving, how do you feel about mechanical telephone answering devices asking for your message after the sound of the beep?

MAKING A LIST

I've been making out lists for years now. Today as I begin my last mile, my agenda for the day forms itself and becomes clear and happy in my mind's eye. Running has surely helped free up my unconscious where all the good ideas are, and let them surface for my attention. Now my new thing to learn is to listen to and trust my new-found source of creativity.

Much of my time management I've learned by osmosis from my Dad. He turned eighty this year and he's still hard at using his gifts of time and talent to their fullest. Here's one paragraph of a letter he sent to me this week:

> "My (business) keeps me busy each day about the right amount. There is too much to do but when one has too much to do he can choose what to do. When I was thirty I made out lists of what had to be done and stuck by it until the list was whittled down. Today I make out the same kind of lists but do what I can each day enjoying every step of the way. Then the next day make out a new list . . ."
>
> — From a personal letter from Gerald R. Prescott, former Bandmaster and Professor at the University of Minnesota

> I have seen the business that God has given to (all) to be busy with.
> — Ecclesiastes 3:10

Do you have enough time to do the things you want and need to do? If your answer is No, why do you suppose that is? Think hard about this for a while. Then find a book on the management of time and put it on your agenda to read this week. (An excellent one to begin with is How to Get Control of Your Time and Your Life by Alan Lakein, Signet Paper Back, 1973.)

WHAT A RACKET!

I'm all noise this morning. The harder I try to be quiet, the more racket I seem to make. At 5:30 a.m. I forget that I have a book on the corner of my desk. Slam! I forget that the door is closed as I come down the stairs. Bam! And "Ouch!" Right on the knee, too; the part of myself I've been protective of lately.

And now when I finally open the back door, one cat runs out and two come in. Son of a gun! They're beginning a fsssst fight. God! If Shirley isn't awake now, she never will be. Sorry, Sweetheart. I'll do better tomorrow.

I recall reading about the monotony and boredom felt so strongly by the men who were kept prisoner during World War II by the Germans. Although Colditz Castle was considered "escape proof," many did make a successful getaway. Because of the "awful sameness" of each day, the men planned escapes endlessly. Also, they were protective of their daily routines. They clung to them with a ferocity that went beyond reason. Those regular routines in their otherwise wretched lives kept them going, it seems.

When Captain "Lulu" Lawton arrived at his section of Colditz, he noticed a note on the door of one of the long time prisoners, from Belgium. It read:

> *"He that blesseth his friend with a loud voice, rising early in the morning, it shall be counted a curse to him."*
>
> (From the Book of Proverbs)

"Lulu" rushed, he said, to his little room to see if it really said that in the Bible.

> — I recall reading about this in:
> *Escape From Colditz*
> by P. R. Reid
> (Lippincott, about 1954)

> He who blesses his neighbor with a
> loud voice, rising early in the morn-
> ing, will be counted as cursing.
> — Proverbs 27:14

What kind of noises do you not like to hear early in the morning?
What kinds do you like to hear?

IT'S GREAT TO BE ALIVE

This evening, as I negotiate Fiechtner Drive along which my friend, a giant rabbit, lives, the sun seems to hang motionless on the horizon, as though the whole clockwork of the universe has finally run down. Then, quite suddenly, it is swallowed by the earth to leave nothing but a cool lavender sky.

I don't very often run at sunset, but when I do, it's almost always a welcome diversion from my usual morning adventure. Today is one of those days. I suppose I've said it before but I feel for sure that there'll never be another sunset to equal this one. Wow! It's great to be alive! All nature is a wonder!

Seymour L. Fishbein, writing about one of my favorite parts of creation, the Boundary Waters Canoe Area of Northern Minnesota and Canada, says:

"We discovered trails around and across the island, crossed beds of feather moss silent to the tread, and piles of dead wood that crunched under every footfall. We lingered in a grove of scraggly, blistered balsams dying of spruce budworm. I touched a blister and fragrant fluid squirted out; in laboratories it's known as Canada balsam, used for cementing specimens to microscope slides . . .

"The lake lies at the core of 230,000 acres of virgin landscape, the largest pristine tract in the Boundary Waters. In the controversies of the 1960s, which burdened the canoe wilderness with compromise, this treasure was preserved. But vast areas of the Boundary Waters' southern perimeter were left open to logging. Conservationists have fought the policy tirelessly, the more so since the perimeter zone includes some 150,000 virgin acres. With time, disturbed terrain may return to wilderness, but in the forest, as elsewhere, virginity is irreplaceable.

> — Seymour L. Fishbein
> "Boundary Waters:
> Canoeing in a Maze"
> *Wilderness USA*
> Edited by Seymour L. Fishbein
> (National Geographic Society,
> 1973) pp. 221-222.

From the rising of the sun to its setting the name of the Lord is to be
praised!
— Psalms 113:3

Can you recall a meaningful encounter with nature, perhaps a sunrise or sunset, that almost made your heart stand still? Close your eyes for a moment and let your unconscious retrieve the scene for you.

BENDING AND WHIRLING

I can feel it in my legs and in my breathing. I am beginning today's run at too great a speed. I need to remind myself of a concept I mentioned in my book, *A Running Commentary*, called "The Warm-up Principle." (p. 10) We need to "ease into" almost all activities. I love the way Satchel Paige, the late baseball warhorse, put it. Someone once asked him for the secret of his amazing stamina. Here's his answer: "I keep moving, like I say, for an hour before I start to pitch. I bend and whirl and loose my muscles up before I ever do throw hard at all."

I think I'll interrupt my run right now and "bend and whirl and loose my muscles up" a little.

> At the West Side YMCA in New York City, where I occasionally run when the winter weather is particularly severe, inexperienced runners sometimes stand beside the track, anxiously watching for an opening. When one appears, they spring into it, sprint two or three laps at top speed, then stop. That's the wrong way to run. First, it isn't nearly enough to do any good. Second . . . in the warm-up you need to raise your body temperature and increase circulation. Those changes don't occur in only a minute or two. They take time — six or eight minutes at the very least. That's why it's a good idea to shuffle along slowly for a while when you first start out. I remember watching John Vitale, one of the country's top distance runners, warming up before a 10,000-meter race in Darien, Connecticut. He was moving so slowly that a toddler would have had little trouble keeping up with him, but later he covered the hilly, winding 6.2-mile course at well under five minutes a mile.
>
> After a few minutes of easy running you'll start to sweat. That's a sign that your warm-up is taking effect and that you're ready to move a little faster.
>
> — James F. Fixx
> *The Complete Book of Running*
> (Random House, 1977), pp. 62-63.

And he stood up to read.
— Luke 4:16

How do you get warmed-up for a run? (Or a game, or a swim, or . . . ?)

A CHILD AGAIN

At least two or three times a week my daily adventure on the roads takes me by Jefferson Elementary, Agassiz Junior High, and South High, the public schools where my children spent some time. Today as I run by the Fargo District Administration Building I recall some words of George Sheehan. "The aim of education," he says, "is to help the child become an adult but at the same time to find the secret of allowing the adult to remain a child." *(Running and Being,* Warner, 1978, p. 80)

I hear you, George. And most clearly when I'm on the path by the Dam, moving at a pace I could hold forever. When my mind is running free, and I'm a child again.

When (Robert Browning) was five, he says, he saw his father reading and asked him what he was reading about. Looking up from his Homer, his father said: "The siege of Troy." "What's a siege?" said the little boy, "and what is Troy?" Now, at this point most fathers would reply: "Troy is a city in Asia, now run off and play with your train." Browning's father was different. He leapt up and began to build Troy, there in the living room. He built a city of tables and chairs. On top he put an armchair for a throne and popped little Robert into it. "There now," he said, "that's Troy, and you're King Priam, and let me see, here's Helen of Troy, beautiful and sleek," and he pointed to the cat beneath the footstool. "Outside, you know the two big dogs in the yard, always trying to get in and catch Helen? They are the fighting kings, Agamemnon and Menelaus, and they are making a siege of Troy so as to capture Helen." And so he told the child as much of the story as could interest him, in just the terms he could understand . . .

And he judges his father a wise teacher for giving him not only an amusement for a day but a possession for all his lifetime.

— Gilbert Highet
The Art of Teaching
(Vintage Books, 1957),
pp. 230-231

> We know that you are a teacher come
> from God.
> — St. John 3:2

Recall one of your early teachers who made learning "live" for you. Write her/him a letter today and say thanks.

THE PIG'S ADVANTAGE

One of the things I really like about running is that each day's excursion has a beginning and an end. There's a measurable finiteness about it. When you're done you know you've accomplished something. Much of my work is hard to pin down that clearly. Most of my projects are in a state of flux, but my daily run is settled.

Today, as I finish up, I find myself with a great big grin on my face. I feel like a dog with two tails!

As human beings we are trapped by our rootage in nature. We are all subject to the forces of aging, sickness, pain, and death. We lack what Big Daddy, in Tennessee Williams' play Cat on a Hot Tin Roof *calls the "pig's advantage" — ignorance of our mortality.* The nature of existential anxiety has been discussed by many thinkers including Soren Kierkegaard, Simone de Beauvoir, Erich Fromm, Paul Tillich, Erik Erikson, Rollo May, Ernest Becker, and Mary Daly. Erikson calls it the "ego chill." Tillich described it as our "heritage of finitude."

. . . Existential anxiety is inherent in our very existence as self-aware creatures. But its influence on us can be either crippling and deadening or creative and enlivening, a stimulus or a barrier to hope and growth, depending on how we respond to it.

— Howard Clinebell
Growth Counseling
(Abingdon, 1979),
pp. 110-111

The years of our life are threescore
and ten, or even by reason of strength
fourscore; yet their span is but toil and
trouble; they are soon gone, and we
fly away.
— Psalms 90:10

What hobbies or work projects give you a sense of well-being because they have a beginning and an end?

THE BEST THINGS IN LIFE ARE FREE

My run takes me down by the river this morning. Spring is coming slowly and almost all the snow is gone. The air is crisp and clear and there is a wondrous quiet about the day. I wonder why I didn't discover this marvelous activity earlier in my life? I wonder why more folks don't take advantage of this most inexpensive of all sports? I encourage everyone I can to at least give it a try. The words of that old song rise out of my unconscious: "The moon belongs to everyone. The best things in life are free." That includes running.

Running's immense popularity is due to its unique advantages. Some of these are:

1) Almost everyone can do it. You don't have to take expensive lessons to be a runner. If you can walk, you probably can work up to running. You can learn what you need to know from magazines, books, and acquaintances who are runners.

2) You can do it almost anywhere. Running doesn't require expensive facilities. You can run in parks, on streets or country roads, in gymnasiums, or on the tracks and running trails found in almost every community.

3) You can do it almost anytime. You don't have to get a team together to run, so you can set your own schedule. Weather doesn't present the same problems and uncertainties that it does in many sports. Running is not a seasonal activity . . . and you can do it in daylight or darkness.

4) It's inexpensive. You don't have to pay to do it, and the only special equipment required is a good pair of running shoes.

> — From "Run For Yourself: An Introduction to Running." A brochure developed by the President's Council on Physical Fitness and Sports. A free copy is available by writing to that Council at Washington, DC 20201.

He makes his sun rise on the evil and
on the good, and sends rain on the
just and on the unjust.
— Matthew 5:45

Name five things in life which are free.

LIVE FOR THE MOMENT

It's April again and that time of the year when Mother Nature begins to liquidate her frozen assets. Only today we have one of those late winter/early spring snows that sets us back a ways. So as I begin my run this morning, it is at a dawn that's still frosty around the edges. As an added image of the incongruity of winter in April I see our deck chair (hauled out of the basement last week) with three inches of snow on it.

Yesterday it was in the fifties and most of the neighborhood kids were out playing. I saw one youngster with roller skates sailing down the sidewalk. I remembered what lousy roller skates we had when I was a kid. They never would stay on and I was forever trying to find a "key." Today they have silent wheels and are built right on to the shoes, like ice skates.

Young people really know how to "live for the moment," don't they? And that's good because it was easier for them to enjoy yesterday not having to think about the forecast for today.

My run on the snow this morning is like playing as a child again. As the ad on TV says, "It doesn't get any better than this!"

Today I want to do things to be doing them, not to be doing something else. I do not want to do things to sell myself on myself. I don't want to do nice things for people so that I will be "nice." I don't want to work to make money, I want to work to work.

Today I don't want to live for, I want to live.
> — Hugh Prather
> *Notes to Myself*
> (Bantam Books, by arrangement with Real People Press, 1976), no page numbers.

> Behold, now is the day of salvation.
> — 2 Corinthians 6:2

What kind of roller skates did you have when you were a kid?

THE YOUNG NURSE

When I was about twelve I broke my elbow trying to jump out of a swing over a green park bench. It was dislocated and it hurt something awful. A stranger drove me home where they called my Dad to come and take me to the hospital. While I waited, scared and sobbing, Lois laid me down on the davenport and brought a cool, wet towel for my forehead. But it was her calm and caring demeanor which brought me the most comfort. I can still recall her strength. I suppose she·was "playing nurse" but was actually being one, too, young as she was.

Twenty eight years later I was at her side when she was hurt. But it was too late. She was already dead. Some days I miss her a lot and cry a little. Like today. You were a great sister, Lois.

All these thoughts come back to me now, as I run by the swings at Island Park, and as I recall that final tragic scene in *Sophie's Choice*.

The passing of time helps, but it cannot fill the empty place. Fell a great tree, and a hole yawns against the skyline. No one ever takes another's place. All of us have a space in existence all our own.

> — Alvin N. Rogness
> *The Book of Comfort*
> (Augsburg, 1979), p. 104

I am reminded of your sincere faith, a faith that dwelt first in your grand-mother Lois.
> — 2 Timothy 1:6

Recall a time when you were injured. Who comes to mind as the person who was most comforting?

WATCHING IT GET DARK

I'm at the Val-Mor Motel at Larimor, North Dakota, on my way back to Fargo after a seminar at Camp Metigoshe. June 14, only one week away from the longest day of the year. It's 9 p.m. and I have just returned from a relaxing thirty-minute run followed by fifteen minutes of easy stretching. Now I'm standing on the lawn watching it get dark. I haven't done this for a long, long time.

As I see the earth and her creatures "settle down," I hear and see many things I normally miss:

- Birds, birds, everywhere birds.
- The sounds of a softball game in the distance.
- Motor bikes revving up and tearing around corners.
- Two men playing horseshoe. Clink.
- The business at the drive-in ice-cream place.
- Eight or nine horses and colts milling around by the barn across the road. Just "appeared."
- A man from India strolling back and forth in front of the motel. Another guest. Looks troubled.
- A tennis match up the road.
- Boys and girls on their bikes hoping for "something to happen."

What a gorgeous, normal, ordinary, wonderful evening in this little corner of the world. What a gift! What a gift! I'm glad I opened it.

I believe that the small moment is the carrier of God's most enduring gifts and that it must not be permitted to slip away unsavored and unappreciated. It is when we fail to take a new look at situations and people close at hand that our dearest relationships suffer. And it is when we mistakenly pursue the unusual and sensational in our quest for fulfillment that we rush past the true meaning of life.

— Gerhard Frost
Blessed Is the Ordinary
(Winston Press, 1980), p. 1

Every good endowment and every
perfect gift is from above . . .
— James 1:17

When was the last time you watched it get dark?

PREJUDICED IN YOUR FAVOR

My Mom used to tell about when I was a kid she had to put a sort of a leash on me when I went along on her store shopping jaunts. I guess I was sort of quick and seemed to disappear a lot. She had a stroke a few years back and can't much "talk things over" anymore. After my run today I was reading Raines and came across these fine words which brought back some old memories for me. I love you, Mom. Thanks for always being so encouraging.

my mother
coming around the corner
seeing me in a fight
with another boy
not knowing whose fault
shouting from half a block away
Give it to him, Bob!
gloriously, blindly prejudiced
in my favor
what it means
to have someone
prejudiced in your favor
unconditional love

my mother
speaking in a contest
whether I won or lost
she thought I was the best
reality problems, pride problems
but what it means
to have someone
think you're the best
loyalty that laid hold deep in me

— Robert A. Raines
Excerpted from "Loyalty That
Laid Hold Deep In Me"
Lord, Could You Make It A
Little Better?
(Word, 1972), p. 49

> And his mother kept all these things
> in her heart.
>
> — Luke 2:51

If you were to describe your Mother in one word, what would it be? Then recall one incident when she seemed to be quite proud of you.

A BRIDGE OF INSTANT RAPPORT

My run this morning takes me by my office and I'm thankful once again for the opportunity to be Director of the FRIENDS Program of North Dakota. After twenty years as a parish pastor I have been given new energy by this mid-life change in vocational energy. Our FRIENDS Program of Lutheran Social Services was started eleven years ago by Jim Merrill and exists to match up people with other people who have experienced similar difficult life situations. I see God at work through these interactions with people who have "been there" in a way that carries much power. While attending a conference at Concordia last week, I was struck by how much Howard Clinebell sounded like he was describing our program. Some words in his book echo what he said in the lecture:

> As a crisis counselor, I never cease to marvel at the way some people turn huge minuses into partial pluses by finding new meaning and strength in even miserable life situations. Within relationships of warmth and trust and caring, many people learn to use their personality muscles in new strengthening ways, taking appropriate action to handle devastating problems and losses constructively. Turning a minus into a partial plus, often involves the discovery, after the worst of a crisis is over, that one's pain can be a bridge of instant rapport with others going through similar losses. Finding out that a crisis has admitted one to a warm bond of mutual caring is like an unexpected gift. (Italics mine)
>
> — Howard Clinebell
> *Growth Counseling*
> (Abingdon, 1979), p. 57.

> If we experience trouble we can pass on to you comfort and spiritual help; for if we ourselves have been comforted we know how to encourage you to endure patiently the same sort of troubles that we have ourselves endured.
>
> — 2 Corinthians 1:6 (Phillips)

"Personality muscles" is a new phrase to me. How do you understand Clinebell's use of this concept?

OVERCOMING "DIN CITY"

I truly enjoy my "running start" of each day by easing out of bed at 5:30 a.m., putting on my sweats, and moving out onto the streets of Fargo. It's as good for my mental well-being as for my physical tuning. Maybe better. I have just returned from a gentle one-hour nine-minute-to-the-mile "therapy" session.

My reading this morning puts me in touch with another minister, from another part of the world, who is an early riser too. But for a different reason. Ever since his seminary days, it has been Archbishop Dom Helder Camara's custom to rise at 2:00 a.m. in order to listen to the voices so frequently drowned out by the daytime noise. Then it is that "God talks to him, nature too, and the human heart." I know, I know. When I run that happens to me.

This Bishop of Brazil writes at that early hour: letters, reports, speeches — and meditations. Here is one of those poetic reflections describing the importance of his habit of more than fifty years:

Among the things to take with me,
I shall not forget you, alarm-clock,
friend fixing the time for my vigils.

Without these,
Din City
would have devoured me.
The child inside me would have died,
having forgotten how to play
and overcome with fear.

Without them,
there would not be
this absolute trust
sealed forever
between us.

— Dom Helder Camara
A Thousand Reasons For
Living
(Fortress, 1981), p. 77.

> I bless the Lord who gives me
>   counsel;
> in the night also my heart instructs
>   me.
> — Psalm 16:7

How do you feel about doing some study and quiet reflection in the wee hours?

FARGO IS ASLEEP

It's just after 5:30 a.m. on the day after Christmas. The snow is falling lightly on Fifth Avenue, on a few parked cars, on roofs and windows, making them glisten. There is no sound as it falls on the pavement. Silently. Fargo is asleep. Quiet. My run feels good.

The Red River is almost frozen over, and by the dam it seems to laugh as it tickles its snowy banks. I'm glad Ruth and Dave got here before St. Paul was snowed in. A newscaster said 35W in the Twin Cities is a "cow path." This is one blizzard that really "winterrupted" the holiday for those south of us. No doubt soon we'll have snowmobiles tearing a rough edge across our winter silence.

The most musical voices of nature are heard only when (we ourselves are) still. It is then that "she speaks a various language." High up on the mountainside, where the Potomac and the Shenandoah mingle their floods to roll together toward the sea, there is a tilting rock known as Jefferson's Rock. According to tradition, it was when he was standing on that rock that Jefferson received inspiration for the description of that grand and beautiful country in his "Notes on Virginia." Far beneath you, toward the south and east, the beautiful Shenandoah flows over shelves of rock. The waters of the Shenandoah make noble music; but if you are speaking or laughing on the rock you cannot hear that music. It is only when you are still that you hear the voice of the river.
— Clarence E. Macartney
Macartney's Illustrations
(Abingdon, 1945), p. 329

For to the snow he says, "Fall on the earth."
— Job 37:6

There is a river whose streams make glad the city of God.
— Psalms 46:4

Close your eyes and recall a peaceful place and moment in your life. Share it with the person next to you.

A '49 FORD

Overpasses are fun to run across and under. Today as I drive west along I-94 I see them from a different perspective. I see these overpasses stapling the highway to the countryside. Quite an image. And moving over this one is an old '49 Ford pick-up. Memories of our beginning days in Fargo and Dave's first car, *his* '49 Ford pick-up, rush in on me. What great times those were! And what a vehicle!

Dave got a little business going, hauling things to the dump for folks. When the city asked us to buy a permit for $100, we asked if he could pay $50 since he was a high-school student and only doing it part time. No deal. We understood. It wouldn't have been fair to the people who make their complete living doing that.

I remember the day it died. It was on Highway 10 as we were returning from a trip to the lake. A fearful sound — a cloud of smoke — and it just absolutely quit. We towed it to Fargo and sold it later "as is."

I wonder what avenue Dave's life would have taken had we paid that fee?

Matt Zaleski sometimes wondered if anyone outside the auto industry realized how little changed, in principle, a final car assembly line was, compared with the days of the first Henry Ford. . . . Nowadays, the final assembly line in any auto plant was unfailingly the portion of the car manufacturing which fascinated visitors most. Usually a mile long, it was visually impressive because an act of creation could be witnessed. Initially, a few steel bars were brought together, then, as if fertilized, they multiplied and grew, taking on familiar shapes like an exposed fetus in a moving womb. The process was slow enough for watchers to assimilate, fast enough to be exciting. The forward movement, like a river, was mostly in straight lines, though occasionally with bends or loops. Among the burgeoning cars, color, shape, size, features, frills, conveyed individuality and sex. Eventually, with the fetus ready for the world, the car dropped on its tires. A moment later an ignition key was turned, an engine sprang to life — as impressive, when first witnessed, as a child's first cry — and a newborn vehicle moved from the assembly line's end under its own power. . . . If old Henry could come back from his grave, Matt thought.

and view a car assembly line of the '70s, he might be amused
at how few basic changes had been made.

> — Arthur Hailey, *Wheels*
> (Doubleday, 1971),
> pp. 317-318

> The driving is like the driving of Jehu
> . . . for he drives furiously.
> — 2 Kings 9:20

My first car was a 1930 Model "A" Ford. What was yours? Does an incident with it come to mind?

FESTINA LENTE

I like to run at a slow pace. It lets me cover more ground, see where I'm going and think about things other than running. It's certainly a cheap, simple, effective antidote to the craziness of modern living. Not everyone can run fast, but almost everyone can run slowly. At least for a little way. I'm surprised more people haven't discovered it. Maybe they think running means speed. But for me, the mental and physical rewards of gentle, everyday running are as great as winning some big race. Today's gentle run is simple exquisite. It matches the Latin words on my T-shirt . . . *Festina Lente*, which, being interpreted means, "Make haste slowly." Good words for me. Maybe for all.

They who have gone slowly all their days; give them garlands and acclaim them great. Their record is deserving of high praise; the voice of duty slowed their eager gait. Seldom spectacular is duty's speed which is maintained the road-length of the years, decided by the daily humdrum need. Flowers for the slow of gait! Give them your cheers! For, when one longs to flee from duty's face, it takes great courage to withstand the urge. The same old road! The uninspiring pace! Over the soul the waves of boredom surge. Here is a record that is hard to beat; never too fast for little humdrum things that must be done for someone else's sake; never too fast to hear a brother's voice; just slow enough as we our journey take, to see the sign-post, Beauty, and rejoice.

— Edward Sidney Kiek
The Battle of Faith
(James Clark and Company,
London, 1938), p. 80

One who believes will not be in haste.
— Isaiah 28:16

What is something you do too fast? How can you slow it down?

THE WOOD PILE

As I leave the house for my morning run, our neighbor's yard light (left on by mistake, no doubt), illuminates our new wood pile. I thought it was a fantastic bargain. A whole cord of wood for only $65. But when we tried to use some that first night we realized it must have been cut just the day before!

If we ever build a house, I'm going to use the kind of wood that was delivered for our fireplace. That way we'll know it will never burn down.

While walking in a New England woods one day, Robert Frost encountered a small bird. His thoughts imagined what the frail creature was thinking until it darted behind a pile of wood. Then came this:

. . . And then there was a pile of wood for which I forgot him and let his little fear carry him off the way I might have gone, without so much as wishing him good-night. He went behind it to make his last stand. It was a cord of maple, cut and split and piled — and measured, four by four by eight. And not another like it could I see. No runner tracks in this year's snow looped near it. And it was older sure than this year's cutting, or even last year's or the year's before. The wood was gray and the bark warping off it and the pile somewhat sunken. Clematis had wound strings round and round it like a bundle. What held it, though, on one side was a tree still growing, and on one a stake and prop, these latter about to fall. I thought that only someone who lived in turning to fresh tasks could so forget his handiwork on which he spent himself, the labor of his ax, and leave it there far from a useful fireplace to warm the frozen swamp as best it could with the slow smokeless burning of decay.

> — From "The Wood-Pile"
> by Robert Frost
> *The Poetry of Robert Frost*
> (Holt, Rinehart and Winston,
> 1969), pp. 101-102

> For lack of wood the fire goes out.
> — Proverbs 26:20

Recall a memory about a wood pile in your life.

MY DAILY RUN

My daily run clears the cobwebs out of my mind and helps me plan my work for the day better. "Our main business," said Carlyle, "is not to see what lies dimly at a distance, but to do what lies clearly at hand." I like that! And what R. Alec Mackenzie espouses speaks to me too: "The heart of time management," he says, "is management of self."

Somehow, my daily run helps put my life in order.

Herman Krannert, as board chairman of Inland Container Corporation, observed, "When I hear a man talk about how hard he works, and how he hasn't taken a vacation in five years, and how seldom he sees his family, I am almost certain that this man will not succeed in the creative aspects of business . . . and . . . most of the important things that have to be done are the result of creative acts."

> — Herman C. Krannert
> "The Time Wasters"
> *The Forum,* Spring, 1969
> Quoted by R. Alec Mackenzie
> in: *The Time Trap*
> (AMACOM, 1972), p. 8

Give us this day our daily bread.
> — St. Matthew 6:11

What activity or process helps clear the cobwebs from your mind?

NO TIME TO BE IN A HURRY

Getting up at 5:30 a.m. really gives me a "running start" on each day. Once in a while, however, I think I'm overdoing it by putting in my five miles *every* morning at this time. Sometimes I even begin to wonder about myself for having made the decision to do this on a regular basis. But getting an early start helps me not have to "rush" through the day. I like that. I need something today, though, that will give me encouragement in my regimen. Some words about John Wesley do that:

> Once when (John Wesley) was asked how he came to have such power, he replied, "For one thing, I have no time to be in a hurry."
>
> Another, was, of course, his flair for system which led him to budget his time. Rising at four in the morning, he was preaching at five. From then until nine or ten at night, every hour-and-a-half had a planned task. In great part, this budgeting of time — rare in the eighteenth century — was what prompted his contemporaries to call him and his likewise methodical disciples "Methodists." At times it was a source of irritation to his friends. Dr. Johnson once complained, "I hate to meet John Wesley. He enchants you with his conversation, and then breaks away to go and visit some old woman. He is always obliged to go at a certain hour. This is very disagreeable to a man who loves to fold his legs and have his talk out, as I do."

— Juliana Lewis
"John Wesley and His Mother,
Susannah"
The Lutheran Journal,
Volume 49, 1982

> For everything there is a season, and
> a time for every matter under heaven.
> — Ecclesiastes 3:1

How do you plan your day? Your week?

RUNNERS AND PILOTS

This morning I see a giant 747 lumbering in for a landing as it floats over Fifth Avenue. It seems to just hang there, heading north into the wind. Runners and pilots think a lot about the wind. We always need to know which way it's blowing. It's a matter of survival. Pilots, for sure. Runners, almost.

Today there's a steady "twenty-knotter" hitting me in the face as I begin. When I began to run, four years ago, I was inside at the Y most of the time. Now I run outside every day, no matter the weather. I like to be in touch with the elements, and besides I see more in the out-of-doors. Like that airplane.

Have you heard the wind names of the world, which are among the least known and most beautiful words? They are truly the heritage of all . . . for they reflect the tongues of history from ancient Cathay to the slang of the United States Army. Consider the dry khamsin of Egypt, reputed to blow sand unceasingly for fifty days; the westerly datoo of the Straits of Gibraltar; the misty waimea of Hawaii; the cool pontias from the Rhone gorges; the chinook of the dry American plains; the sudden violent williwaw of Alaska and Magellan's Strait; the biting black buran of Russia; . . . the playful vento coado which whistles through the crannies in hillside hovels of Portugal; . . . the dainty feh of Shanghai; the whirling tsumuji of Japan; the vindictive rok of Iceland; the refreshing imbat off the blue Mediterranean; the ruthless helm wind of Cumberland which uproots turnips in the field.

> — Guy Murchie
> *Song of the Sky*
> (Houghton Mifflin, 1954),
> p. 130

And God made a wind blow over the
earth . . .
> — Genesis 8:1

What is the strongest wind you have ever experienced?

OUR THOUGHTS ARE HANDED TO US

It takes me a heck of a while to drive anyplace these days, as I have to pull over, stop and write quite often. Otherwise the thoughts that are "handed to me" get lost. Or dropped.

As I finish writing this note, I look up and see a sign which says:

> Clark Salyer
> National Wildlife
> Refuge

I'm in the northern part of Central North Dakota on my way to Westhope.

> *The greater part of what emerges into consciousness comes from the unconscious. We do very little "thinking"; rather,* our thoughts are handed to us. *The ideas, impulses, effects, emotions, imaginary events, and conversations that we call fantasies stream through us out of their source in the unconscious. This is undirected thinking. It may be especially conspicuous to us, for instance, if we pay attention to what crosses our minds as we take a shower, or what we find ourselves dwelling upon when we are driving alone on the freeway. Most people pay no attention to the source of the stream of consciousness and so they miss the presence of the unconscious in their lives. To keep a journal is to begin to reverse this state of negligence and take into account the unseen source of our psychic life.*
> — John A. Sanford
> *Healing and Wholeness*
> (Paulist Press, 1977),
> pp. 123-124

> An angel of the Lord appeared to him
> in a dream . . .
> — Matthew 1:20

How do you feel about "hunches?" Have you ever acted on one that turned out well and surprised you?

WORDS OF CHEER

"You're lookin' good!" An encourager shouts that greeting to me as I move past his house. He's in his pajamas reaching out of his half-open door for the morning paper. "Thanks, neighbor," I call back.

I love to hear words of cheer. I need to. There will be plenty of times without them. I'm going to accept and absorb them today, like a warm cup of coffee. "You're lookin' good," is a compliment, and it needs to be savored.

True, all children need to experience their competence to build self-respect. But each child needs to feel that his person is cherished regardless of his competence. Successful performances build the sense of worthwhileness; being cherished as a person nurtures the feelings of being loved. Every child needs to feel both loved and worthwhile. But lovability must not be tied to worthwhile performance. The more lovable any child feels, however, the more likely he is to perform in satisfactory ways, for then he likes himself.

> — Dorothy Corkille Briggs
> *Your Child's Self-Esteem*
> (Doubleday and Co., 1970)
> Quoted in *100 Ways to Enhance Self-Concept in the Classroom,* by Jack Canfield and Harold C. Wells (Prentice Hall, 1976), p. 49

A word fitly spoken is like apples of gold in a setting of silver.
> — Proverbs 25:11

Recall the last time you received a compliment. How did you accept it?

A COLD MORNING

I never do run very fast. About nine minutes for a mile during my daily fix. But today I'm even slower, because *it's cold!* Twenty below maybe. As I round the corner by the big apartment complex I see many automobile hoods yawning on this freezing morning, waiting to be jump started.

Only a short distance into my morning run my feet still only slap and stomp at the asphalt. I feel like that teammate of his Dizzy Dean commented on: "He runs too long in one place. He's gotta lot of up 'n' down, but not much forward."

Runner B trains on LSD. (Long, slow, distance) His run begins as soon as he gets out of bed and gets on his shoes and shorts. Out the door he goes and down the street. He's free to go where his legs take him. Unhurried, unworried. Sidewalks, streets, parks, golf courses, country roads, even an occasional tract, all are in abundant supply. The variety is vast. Training is never quite the same. No complicated training equations fill his head. It's an hour or so full of running, and one which he usually finishes feeling fresher, more awake than when he stumbled out.

> — Joe Henderson
> *Long Slow Distance: The Humane Way to Train*
> (Tafnews Press, 1969), p. 14

> Again I saw that under the sun the
> race is not to the swift . . .
> — Ecclesiastes 9:11

If you have not run for a while, why not do it today? Slowly . . . for one block at least.

POETRY

Breakfast follows my morning run, and that is followed lately by Shirley and me reading some poetry by Robert Frost. Today when I read these surprisingly forceful words I shouted out loud, "Wow!"

"Steel-bright June-grass,
and blackening heads of clover."*

This is from his piece called "The Exposed Nest" and helps me understand Emily Dickinson's response to the question someone put to her, "What is good poetry? She answered something like, "I can't tell you, but if you feel like it's taking off the top of your head as you read it, then that's great poetry."

A technique that works for groups from junior high school through adult levels involves training students' emotional responses through the use of poetry. Better than any other form of writing, poetry combines ideas with emotion. In poetry the author attempts to create in language a situation that will recreate a particular response in the reader. Unfortunately, too many poor teachers of English have been loose for too long, and poetry has become for many students or former students a dry, overly complicated group of words with a sing songy rhyme whose purpose is to create problems for readers.

If you are in that group, trust me! Poetry is worth another try. Read correctly, poetry makes the world more alive and vibrant, more exciting and revealing than it has been before.

— Ryan LaHurd
"Jolting Effie's Gingerbread"
Article in "Learning With"
Magazine
January, 1978, p. 3

---

* *The Poetry of Robert Frost*, Edited by Edward Connery Lathem (Holt, Rinehart and Winston, 1969), p. 109.

. . . for
"In him we live and move and
   have our being";
as even some of your poets
      have said,
   "For we are indeed his off-
      spring."
                        — Acts 17:28

What is one of your favorite poems? Do you have it memorized? If not, do so this week.

HELLO

My run takes me along University Drive this morning and almost everyone is returning my hello. I love that. One of the things I recall about my Dad is that he used to say hello to everyone. He was Professor of Music Education at the University of Minnesota and Director of the Concert and Marching Bands. It didn't matter if it was Dimitri Mitropoulos or John Smith, when Dad passed someone in the hall of the Northrup Memorial Auditorium building it was always "Hello." And he put his heart into it. It was his "Shalom."

He's retired from teaching now and lives in Florida. I bet he's still brightening up our world with his "hellos!"

The only other person I remember saying hello that much is "Pinky" Lofgren from our class of '48 at Marshall High.

The Hebrew word shalom is a word with positive connotations. Freely translated it refers to the existence of a creative force for good throughout the world. Shalom denotes a sense of completeness, a sense of fulfillment, a sense of wholeness, a sense of being at one with oneself.
> — Rabbi Arthur S. Hollander
> as quoted in
> *The Quotable American Rabbis*
> (Droke House, 1967), p. 189

And he said, Peace be to you, fear not.
> — Genesis 43:23 (KJV)

And behold, Jesus met them and said, "Hail!"
> — Matthew 28:9 (RSV)

It has been stated that "we ought to be kind, since most people we meet are fighting a tough battle." Do you agree? Can a simple greeting like "Hello" change much?

A FRAGILE PRIZE

Looking at the 0:49 40 on my digital watch I'm beaming and proud of myself. 10-K in under fifty minutes. It's been a goal of mine for quite a while.

This little timepiece (my friend, Edie, calls it "one of those rubber watches") is one of the greatest inventions in the history of running. It not only helps you improve your running but it also gives an accurate record of your results. Trouble is, when I run again tomorrow, I'll know how fragile my prize is because the time will come to reset the digits, to wipe away the old result and start putting some new numbers on the dial. And I do that by one quick push of the button.

The racing part of running gives me good perspective on what is important. The results and reward of a "good race" go quickly, but the sustained effect of my daily training (90% of all my running) helps me enjoy each moment of my existence.

Yesterday is past.
Tomorrow is not yet.
So live today.

— Reuben K. Youngdahl

This is the day which the Lord has
made;
let us rejoice and be glad in it.
— Psalm 118-24

I had 1:40 (an hour and forty minutes) on my watch the other day. And I was proud of that long workout. But while dingin' around with the "mode selection" buttons I accidentally erased it. I had wanted to keep it registered to remind me of my super effort. Have you ever "erased" something you really wanted to keep? (A letter thrown away? A magazine article you were going to save forever? _____?)

ALL THOSE T-SHIRTS

It's a rainy fourth of July. Nice day to be home "catching up" on a few projects. One of those projects is to lay out all my T-shirts. They've been accumulating over the years and I've never seen them all together. Wow! Such memories from these prizes and gifts. Super Grandpa, Red River Run, Hug Therapist, Lake Agassiz Pacers, I'm Suzy's Dad, Sal Si Puede, International Runner, Festina Lente, 916 Vo Tech, Simul Justus et Peccator, U.S. Navy, Hang Loose-Hawaii and Boundary Waters Chase. And about fifteen more. I may be slow, but by God I'm interesting reading!

Where would long distance runners be without t-shirts? I have collected so many t-shirts at races that I rarely buy under-shirts at the store. It is embarrassing to be seen at parties wearing a Brooks Brothers three-piece suit, Gucci loafers, silk tie, gold pin, the whole bit, and have "Road Runners Track Club" visible under your shirt. If you ever hear of any races where they give plain white t-shirts for prizes, mail me an entry blank.
— Hal Higdon
Beginner's Running Guide
(World Publications, 1978),
p. 120

To each and all of them
he gave festal garments . . .
— Genesis 45:22

What does your favorite T-shirt say?

THE LOST DATEBOOK

For years I have joked about the fact that if I ever lost my calendar/datebook I'd have to leave off being a pastor and go into another vocation. My datebook is that important to me.

Well, it finally happened! While conducting a funeral last Friday at Iver's Funeral Home, someone walked off with my briefcase which was, where I always leave it, in the backroom. In it were my sermon notes for the next Sunday, four books, one of my favorite Bibles, papers . . . and my calendar/datebook.

After all the funeral home folks and I searched high and low, I called the police and reported it missing. When they came I described the contents. One of the detectives said, "Yes, and was there anything of *real* value in it?"

Here are two ads I placed in the Fargo Forum:

HELP! My calendar/datebook has been taken. If you have an appointment with me for anytime this summer please drop me a note with the date and time. Thanks, friends! Roger Prescott, 670 4th Ave., N. Fgo.

REWARD! Would the person who must have inadvertently carried away my briefcase from Ivers Funeral Home please return it? Especially needed are my calendar/datebook and sermon notes. Some of my favorite books were in it too! People have often said "He doesn't know if he's coming or going", but now without my calendar/datebook it's really true. PLEASE return my stuff! No questions asked. Rev. Roger Prescott, St. Mark's Church, 670 4th Ave. N., Fgo. 235-5591, 293-1925.

The Forum
Fargo-Moorhead,
May 28, 1980, p. 27

He shall restore what he took . . . or
the lost thing which he found.
— Leviticus 6:4

Did you ever lose your calendar/datebook? How did you deal with that loss? If you haven't lost one, what do you think you'd do if you did?

MIDDLE AGE FORGETFULNESS

As I run under the bridge on Main Avenue during my daily adventure along the river, I spot a car overhead that has some kind of object on its top I know doesn't belong there. Forgotten, no doubt, by the driver after placing it there while he negotiated the door.

Last time I did that I was lucky. It was only a sack of garbage. Was I embarrassed when Bob brought it into the office and said, "Rog, you left this on top of your car." In the past I haven't been that lucky. One time it was a jar of Gatorade. Smashed and spilled as I rounded the first corner. Another day it was my briefcase. Thank God for the people who make things strong. I wonder if it's true that I'm doing this more often than before?

I turned forty a while ago
and came dribbling out of the locker room
ready to start the second half
glancing up at the scoreboard
I saw that we were behind 7 to 84
and it came to me then we ain't gonna win
and considering the score
I'm beginning to be damn glad
this particular game ain't gonna go on forever.

But don't take this to mean I'm ready
for the showers
take it to mean I'm probably gonna play
one helluva second half

I told this to some kids in the court
next to mine and they laughed
but I don't think they understood how could they
playing in the first quarter only one point behind
　　　　　　　　　　　　— Ric Masten
　　　　　　　　　　　　The Second Half
　　　　　　　　　　　　The Deserted Rooster
　　　　　　　　　　　　(Sunflower Ink, 1982), p. 7.

Moses was a hundred and twenty
years old when he died; his eye was
not dim, nor his natural force abated.
— Deuteronomy 34:7

As age creeps up on you, how do you notice that is so?

NOTHING IS REALLY FRIGHTENING

Gertrude Stein said a lot of nifty things. And I just love something I read recently. Only she could have said, "Considering how dangerous everything is, nothing is really frightening."

Isn't that great! Isn't that fine! Gives a person a whole new perspective. Running *can be* dangerous, especially if you push too hard or too close to traffic. But it isn't very often frightening. Even when I'm worried about my iliotibial bands or Achilles tendons. (No, those aren't rock groups!)

In fact even when I do overdo it (and I always do), by preparing for and running a marathon or half-marathon, I console myself with these words of another grand lady. "Too much of a good thing," said Mae West, "can be wonderful!"

> *The Church must not be afraid to try some experiments which may not show any statistical result. This can be carried too far, but there must be places where we move into society with no hope of advancing the Church as an institution. On this path there will be many failures and we should expect them. The Christian minister who is doing his (or her) job always has some far-out experiments going on in the hopes that (they) may stumble on something to break the defences of a secular society.*
>
> — Gerald Kennedy, *The Seven Worlds of the Minister* (Harper and Row, 1968), p. 140

> Say to those who are of a fearful heart, "Be strong, fear not!"
> — Isaiah 35:4

If you knew you couldn't fail, what is something you would like to try?

ONLY THREE THINGS EVER SCARED ME

Fargo's Country Club property bumps up against Riverside Cemetery. Two naturally beautiful and well-kept developments. Right where they meet is one of the "turn-around" points for one of my forty-five-minute runs. Over the past twelve years I've spent time at both these spots.

This morning it is so beautiful out, my mind is turning to many golf courses and many enjoyable hours spent on them. And just yesterday I heard this on the radio. I became so nostalgic that I stopped the car and wrote it out as closely as I could. Let me share this piece with you. It's the end of an era:

> Sam Snead is retiring from golf this year, after fifty years on the tour. He is seventy-one. His swing is still as smooth as ever but he's lost depth perception in one eye. He hasn't lost his old wit, however, as witnessed by his words at a recent banquet honoring his many contributions to the game. "Only three things about golf ever scared me," he drawled. "Lightning; downhill putts; and Ben Hogan!"

So long Sam. Thanks for all the inspiration and instruction you have given us all. During your retirement, may the wind be mostly at your back.

> For everything there is a season, and
> a time for every matter under heaven:
> . . . a time to seek, and a time to lose;
> a time to keep, and a time to cast
> away.
> — Ecclesiastes 3:1, 6

Beginning with Arnold Palmer, Babe Didrikson Zaharias and Gene Littler, call to mind as many of the recent and old-time golf greats as you can think of.

BIRDS

Some days it's dogs. Other mornings it's cats. But today I see birds everywhere. Before I began running each day I don't think I ever *really* noticed the birds. But I do now. And how! Such beauty and tenderness they bring to our world. It's my judgment that my daily five has heightened my consciousness to all things. How about you? Been noticing any birds lately?

I never noticed the birds for the first forty years or so of my life . . . I was too busy trying to make it, fulfilling big production quotas for the Lord, the Church, and maybe chiefly for myself. There was little time for walking beside still waters, lifting up my eyes to the hills, or noticing the birds. I neglected the natural. I lost the sense of my creatureliness, and so forfeited nature's healing of mind and body. How sweet it is to notice the birds! I feel a freshening of quietness and confidence, a gracious restoration of strength. And I am beginning to accept, a little, my dying and my living as a loved creature.

> — Robert A. Raines
> *Living the Questions*
> (Word Books, 1976),
> pp. 16-17

Look at the birds of the air . . .
— Matthew 6:26

What are some of the varieties of birds you can recall seeing?

PUDDLES

It's spring again for sure. There are puddles with ice on them everywhere. I have to be careful because some of them don't hold me, and I break through and get my feet wet. This is indeed the time of year when "mother nature" begins to liquidate her frozen assets.

I recall one spring in Minneapolis. I was about ten or eleven, I guess. Tower Hill had a low spot at its base, on the other side. One year some water formed there and then froze over. As a young lad I had to "try it out." Mom was both angry and frightened when I came home all "sopping" wet, snowsuit, overshoes and all. I think that puddle was two or three feet deep!

I wish I were
a humble puddle
that would reflect the sky!

— Dom Helder Camara
A Thousand Reasons for Living
(Fortress Press, 1981), p. 19

He gives snow like wool . . .
He casts forth his ice like morsels . . .
He sends forth his word, and melts
them.

— Psalm 147:16-18

Do you recall an incident with a puddle from your youth?

THE UNFAIR DISTRIBUTION OF SUFFERING

As I run by the old brown house, I wonder how this day will be for the folks who live there? Since Jim took his life a couple of years ago, they've had more than their share of trouble and hurt. Why have I been so lucky in my life? Why have they had such heavy burdens? Why do bad things happen to good and decent people? Why? Why? Why?

There is only one question which really matters: why do bad things happen to good people? All other theological conversation is intellectually diverting; somewhat like doing the crossword puzzle in the Sunday paper and feeling very satisfied when you have made the words fit; but ultimately without the capacity to reach people where they really care. Virtually every meaningful conversation I have ever had with people on the subject of God and religion has either started with this question, or gotten around to it before long. Not only the troubled man or woman who has just come from a discouraging diagnosis at the doctor's office, but the college student who tells me that he has decided there is no God, or the total stranger who comes up to me at a party just when I am ready to ask the hostess for my coat, and says, "I hear you're a rabbi; how can you believe that . . . " — they all have one thing in common. They are all troubled by the unfair distribution of suffering in the world.

> — Harold S. Kushner, *When Bad Things Happen to Good People* (Schocken Books, 1981), p. 6

"Where were you when I laid the foundation of the earth? Tell me, if you have understanding."
— Job 38:4

Can you think of an instance when a very bad thing happened to a person you know, and you wondered why?

TWO CAN

There they are again. That older couple walking hand in hand. They always ignore me unless I run right by them. They are polite and say hello. But it's obvious to me they are caught up in their own togetherness. That's great. As Shirley and I approach our thirtieth anniversary (just two days after Suzy and Tod's wedding), I'm thankful for her faithful partnership, lo these many years.

Maybe one of the most beautiful things ever said about marriage was said by that notable philosopher Humpty Dumpty, in *Alice Through the Looking Glass*. Humpty is reproaching Alice for her rate of growth:

> "I never ask advice about growing," Alice said indignantly.
> "Too proud?" (Humpty Dumpty) inquired.
> Alice felt even more indignant at this suggestion. "I mean," she said, "that one cannot help growing old."
> "One can't, perhaps," said Humpty Dumpty, "but two can."

> — Lewis Carroll
> *Through the Looking Glass*
> (New American Library, 1960),
> p. 184 (*Through the Looking Glass* was originally published between 1855 and 1871)

. . . and they become one flesh.
— Genesis 2:24

Someone, possibly Gertrude Stein, said: "We are all the same age on the inside. What do you understand her to mean by that? And what did Humpty Dumpty mean by "two can?"

DAYS AWAY

Even great and joyous things can't be sustained too regularly. I love to run so much that it's hard for me to take days away from it. And yet . . . and yet I know my body is telling me to take it easy. Six days ago I completed the Manitoba Half-Marathon and my Achilles tendon is asking for rest. Nothing serious, but enough so that practical sense says I need a couple of days' vacation from running. Today instead of running, I'm up at my usual time and digging dandelions in the yard . . . and stretching a little. God!, but I am compulsive, aren't I?

If days off must be taken from extra things we love and are nourished by, how much more ought we have days away from our main work? I'm speaking to myself here . . . and to all my colleagues in the ministry . . . and all other vocations which "have no end to the work" to them.

> *It is important that the day off (or two days off) be kept sacred, with none of the usual activities, because the purpose of such a day is to enter into a new state of consciousness. By removing yourself from your usual surroundings and tasks you allow a new consciousness to take shape. But it is like going swimming — you need to get all the way into the water. If the day is broken up by some official task, the new kind of consciousness that is beginning to develop is broken. That is why just a few hours off here and there do not renew us sufficiently. It takes longer than that for the invisible threads that connect us to our work to be relaxed so that new thoughts, new moods, new experiences, can find their way in.*
> — John A. Sanford
> *Ministry Burnout*
> (Paulist Press, 1982), p. 19

> "Come away by yourselves to a lonely place, and rest a while."
> — Jesus
> St. Mark 6:31

Do you take at least one full day off each week? Do you ever, on that day, break it up by some official task? (Like, "Just this one phone call," or "I'm going to stop by the office just for a minute.")

THE GREAT LEVELER

A foot race is a great "leveler." No one asks what your station in life is. What you do for a living. Or about your accomplishments. Only, "Nice race, man!" Or "Way to go!" Maybe a "How'd you do?" Unless I know about the participants before the race, I never think to ask about their lives. Such camaraderie in running!

Today a friend told me about the time a pastor first arrived at a new parish. At an after-church reception one of the "pillars" of the congregation seized his arm and said, "Come along with me. I want you to meet the right people." The wise pastor handled that sad situation well by saying, "I want to meet *all* the people."

> *. . . The theologians are taking a hard look at the thought that we must become as little children to enter the Kingdom. If so, there is nothing more characteristic about children than their love of play. No one comes into this world a Puritan. If there is anything children care less about, it is work and money and power and what we call achievement.*
>
> *We watch and envy as they answer the call, "Come and play."*
>
> — George Sheehan, M.D.
> *Running and Being*
> (Warner Books, 1978), p. 72

> And the streets of the city shall be full
> of boys and girls playing in its streets.
> — Zechariah 8:5

> . . . All have sinned and fall short of
> the glory of God.
> — Romans 3:23

Running is a form of adults, "playing together." What are some other ways? What's your favorite?

AN ANNOUNCEMENT OF REALITY

Sometimes when I run it's dark the whole time, and the world seems almost unreal. It's like that this October morning. So now, after my daily fix, as I'm driving towards a meeting in Minneapolis, it's good for my soul to see the silhouette of this small midwestern town's water-tower (Frazee, Minnesota) just before sunrise. A crisp, clear, and focused announcement of reality.

The heavenly guest
is at the door.

The other day, at dawn,
for just a moment,
the lines were clear.

I saw.

Today they blur again,
but then, for a little while,
I saw, I really did.

And, thank God,
I'll see again.

> — Gerhard Frost
> *Kept Moments*
> (Winston, 1982), p. 75

> And he shewed me a pure river of
> water of life, clear as crystal . . .
> — Revelation 22:1 (KJV)

What helps you see things crisp and clear?

OLDER RUNNERS

I'm feeling bushed today. And I haven't run all that far. Must be getting old. I probably just need to lighten up a little for a while. Running is one sport that we "older" people can do for a long time. Here's a story about an "older" runner that lifts my heart today:

> *The leader of the over-fifty runners in the 1979 Boston and New York City marathons was a 130-pound producer of television documentaries named Don Dixon, who ran 2:39 and 2:43, respectively. He was fifty-one years old for the first race, fifty-two for the second . . .*
>
> *Back in the 1940s Dixon ran for his high school cross-country team. He admits, however, that he wasn't very good at it. "Even on my best day," he says, "I often came in last." After graduation he gave up running and didn't take the sport up again until he was almost forty. Waiting for a handball court at a YMCA one day, he decided to pass the time by circling the track a few times. "One day," he says, "I ran three miles. It was the farthest I had ever gone. I felt very satisfied." On a whim Dixon entered the 1971 Yonkers Marathon, which passes not far from his home in Hastings-on-Hudson, New York. He finished in 3:35. Later the same year he ran the New York City Marathon. This time he ran a 3:25. Encouraged, he started working out harder. In his eleventh marathon, the Earth Day on Long Island, he finally broke three hours.*
>
> — James F. Fixx
> *Jim Fixx's Second Book of Running* (Random House, 1978), pp. 108-109

> They still bring forth fruit in old age,
> they are ever full of sap and green . . .
> — Psalm 92:14

What is the farthest you have ever run?

FEELINGS

I like running in different places. Today I'm in Moline, Illinois. That Church over there looks like Grace Lutheran in southeast Minneapolis. Reminds me of the time my Mom took me there to see and hear Frank Laubach. I don't recall anything he said during his sermon (I was about twelve or so), but I do remember shaking his hand on the way out. He had a firm grip, looked me right in the eye and said, "Young man! Hit the world hard!"

The other day I talked with Gerhard Frost and had a chance to tell him how much I was nourished by his writing. Especially his reminiscences of long ago times. Then he said something that sticks with me still. "The things we remember from our long ago past are always 'feeling' things. We may not remember the date or the circumstances, but we remember the 'feelings'." Today I remember with "feeling" my encounter with Frank Laubach.

I saw him only once,
my traveling companion on our way to Boston,
back in the railroad's glory days.
We were both young then;
not so today, but I remember him for something that he said.

He was a ready talker with not much room for silence.
For hours we moved from this to that
in easy-to-be-forgotten repartee,
but this, of all he said, remains with me:
"I always talk to old people."

If I could see him now I'd thank him and I'd say
how many times I've recalled,
even practiced, what he said.
Good sense, to speak to those
who've been there, to listen and not regret.
> — Gerhard Frost
> *Kept Moments*
> (Winston, 1982), p. 52

> And Peter remembered the sayings of Jesus.
> — Matthew 26:75

Recall one incident that happened when you were just a kid. What kind of feelings go along with it?

INSPIRED TO RUN

"Hi, Rog. Jim Hicks here. Nothing important. Well, yes, as a matter of fact, it's very important." These were the words that came over the phone when I picked it up just moments ago. "Just wanted you to know that your book inspired me to run today. I just got back. Ran three quarters of a mile, stretched about fifteen minutes and then walked a mile. I feel great."

He thinks *he* feels great. He ought to know that I do too because that's one of the purposes of my writing; to get people to thinking about and beginning to do something good for themselves. Like running.

Hang in there, Jim. And be careful. Your whole life could take a new turn.

And to think at first the ringing of the phone was an irritation.

> *Beginning makes the mind*
> *grow heated:*
> *When you start*
> *the task's completed.*
>
> — Goethe (Paraphrased)

> . . . And this is only the beginning of
> what they will do; and nothing that
> they propose to do will now be im-
> possible for them.
>
> — Genesis 11:6

Why do you suppose it is so hard to begin doing some things, and so easy to finish them? What is one such activity for you?

AFTER EVERYTHING WAS
SUPPOSED TO BE OVER

I am quaffing orange slices and cups of Pepsi like they're going out of style! What a tremendous feeling to have just completed the Manitoba Half Marathon. In the recovery area they have provided every kind of refreshment for these many tired bodies. What a thrill to mingle with all these athletes as they laugh and talk and recall their race! There's a camaraderie here that I haven't felt since my days in the Marine Corps. I like this Half Marathon. I'm not fast enough for the shorter races and I don't seem to be able to make the time to train for a full marathon. I think I've found my distance. I believe we are all, as Dr. George Sheehan says, "an experiment of one." And it's good to tarry here with all these other researchers.

I read somewhere that a man who had recently exerted himself tremendously (maybe in a big race) said: "I felt fine the next day, until I started walking around. Then my body tried to kill me!" Such may tomorrow be, but for the moment, all is well. How really good it is to be able to savor this unique time and place.

Robert Frost speaks about the time he missed a train after a meeting "and the evening was added to the afternoon." During this time he talked with a young Ph.D. of Harvard 1921 who believed in suicide as the only noble death. He says:

"Now if I hadn't formed the habit of staying round after everything was supposed to be over, you can see what I would have missed."

— Robert Frost,
The Years of Triumph,
1915-1938 by Lawrence
Thompson, (Holt, Rinehart,
Winston, 1970), p. 250

. . . They besought him that he would
tarry with them.
-- St. John 4:40 (KJV)

How do you feel about "hanging around" after an event or meeting?

GUARANTEED HIERARCHICAL PRIVILEGES

I'm glad I discovered running in my middle years because it was the trigger for the writing I now do. And my writing has led to more speaking engagements and "playshops." (I never did like the name "workshop." Sounds like too much drudgery.) The extra income from my writing has made the difference between an adequate and a comfortable income.

What a liberating feeling to be able to have a diversity of ways to earn a living.

I'm not running very far this morning because my body is still recovering after the Manitoba Half Marathon. I miss the feeling of well-being that comes from a leisurely long run.

A few persons who are in their middle-age years maintain a diversity of ways of earning a living. They are sufficiently nonchalant about getting both prestigious offices and the perquisites of such offices that their lives have remained at base simple and free of a lot of trappings. They can live on the periphery by the "weight of their being" as persons and not by reason of the particular "connections," "platforms," or "positions" they have. They have not permitted themselves to become "entangled" in what Aldous Huxley called "guaranteed" hierarchical privileges. The human spirit was created for this kind of freedom. The purpose of redemption is to restore that kind of freedom if it has been lost.

> — Wayne E. Oates
> *Workaholics, Make Laziness Work for You*
> (Doubleday, 1978), p. 41

For to the one who has will more be given, and that one will have abundance . . .
> — St. Matthew 13:12

Besides the way you are now earning a living, how else would you like to make or receive some money?

SELF ESTEEM

"I never met a person," said one of my friends recently, "who had a self-esteem that was too high." I second the motion.

My running brings a new sense of feeling good about myself. I'm convinced we all need that. As I glide along today I'm proud of my middle-aged self for doing something everyday for just myself alone. Especially when it's not immoral, illegal or fattening. Besides, it's almost free.

Did you ever notice how children have a natural acceptance of themselves . . . until the "adult" world makes them "grow up"?

Bil Keane, the cartoonist, has a strip he calls "The Family Circle." In one of his offerings he depicts a small boy waiting in line at a drinking fountain in a school. Obviously flushed and excited from much play at recess, he is saying to the one drinking in front of him, "Hurry up! Hurry up! I've got to get back out there and let them enjoy me some more!"

> . . . For God made (humanity) in his own image.
> — Genesis 9:6

What activity do you do that brings you a better feeling about yourself?

A GREAT TIME WAS HAD BY ALL

As we wait for the official results, it's fun to "mill around" after a race. There were 249 finishers in this one, The Boundry Waters Chase. All seemed euphoric.

I still get the usual question, "How'd you do, Rog?" And I still love to give my usual answer. "How'd I do? Well, I didn't get lost. I finished. and I had a great time!"

Hope I'll be able to say that about my life when I am breathing my last. I hope we all can.

> Time and experience revealed to me that life was a trip, not a goal. That often one became so fixed on the end that (they) totally missed life along the way, and found, only too late, that when (they) had scaled the mountain there was only another mountain, and another, and another. What a pity that (they) had never stopped long enough to breathe the new, clean, fresh air and admire the spectacular view. I had to question: If life is a continual trip, does it matter if one ever "gets" anywhere?
>
> — Leo Buscaglia
> The Way of the Bull
> (Charles B. Slack, 1973) p. x.

> I came that they may have life, and have it abundantly.
> — St. John 10:10

Do you agree with Leo Buscaglia that "life is a trip, not a goal?" Why?

A HAPPY GASP

We had a beautiful snowfall last night. As I run by that gorgeous condominium just on the south edge of Island Park, I hear a "scrape-scrape-scrape." I look to see where it's coming from and I see an old man shoveling the driveway. He sees me just as I see him and he utters what I could only describe as a "happy gasp." Seems glad to see me. I call to him, "What a great day this is!" He answers with vigor, "How far do you run?" "About five miles," I call over my shoulder. "Great," he says, "Have a wonderful day!" He's still shouting good things to me as I run out of range. "I hope you . . . " I wonder what those last words were? I wonder about his "story."

In the Inn of the world there is room for everyone. To turn your back on even one person, for whatever reason, is to run the risk of losing the central piece of your jigsaw puzzle.
— Leo Buscaglia
The Way of the Bull
(Charles B. Slack, 1973), p. 79

Are not two sparrows sold for a penny? And not one of them will fall to the ground without your Father's will. But even the hairs of your head are all numbered. Fear not, therefore; you are of more value than many sparrows.
— St. Matthew 10:29-31

Do you think of your love for God primarily in horizontal or vertical terms? If you are with someone now, talk about that a little bit.

A SORT OF A PRAYER

In a few days I'll be running in the Manitoba Half Marathon so my workout today is very light. All the books say to taper off a few days before a big race. Well, I'm surprised to say I miss that daily forty-five minutes on the road. I feel so strong and full of running that it's hard to go only a couple of miles. Yet concentrating on listening to the experience of many people is important. I think it's a sort of prayer.

The event will be Sunday in Winnipeg so Shirley and I are going a few days early and make a little vacation out of it. Tony and Sharon are going too so we'll have a real party. We look forward to dining at Churchill's and I'll have a chance to buy another snazzy necktie at The Hudson Bay or Eaton's.

The whole weekend is going to be an experience in paying attention to life. To me, these days, that's real conversation with God.

Let us pray.

Prayer is the outward yearning of my inward being. Whenever I am really seeing, hearing, touching, smelling, remembering, hoping with all my heart, I am praying. Some of us may think of God as a person out there, listening, caring, responding. Some of us may think of God as the power and spirit that holds all things together, sustaining, enabling, embracing. We try to name the silence and to see the face of the darkness, for we do not want to pour out our yearning into chaos or nothingness. So we reach into the silence and listen to the darkness and try to trust the source of all that is and remember to be amazed that there is something instead of nothing.

— Robert A. Raines, *Lord, Could
You Make It a Little Better?*
(Word Books, 1972) p. 14

And in praying do not heap up empty
phrases . . .
— St. Matthew 6:7

Kevin Coughlin says that "Prayer is paying attention to our every-day lives." Discuss that a little bit. Do you agree? Disagree? What forms of prayer are the most natural expressions for you?

SENTENCES THAT SING

Might as well get it out into the open. I like to write almost as much as I like to run. At least it's enjoyable to "have written." Writing helps me express my feelings. Putting words on paper by way of my old Royal clears the corners of my mind and leaves freshness for new growth. Someone said the art of writing begins with "placing the seat of the pants on the seat of the chair." Put another way Joe Henderson says "Good writing is the product of starting with the first word and putting down whatever comes after that." We do a lot of other things for sheer enjoyment (golfing, stamp collecting, acting in community plays, fishing), so why not writing? I'm an advocate of writing just for fun. That's when my best writing comes. If it happens to be publishable, it's incidental (Well, almost). Publishing came slowly for me. An article in the Christian Ministry in 1974. One in Golf Magazine in 1977. Another in the Christian Ministry in 1981. My first book in 1981. Then two in 1983. Now almost one article and one book a year. I'm in high gear and I love it.

As I finish this morning's run. I can hardly wait to get up to my room and finish today's piece. Part of this day's plan is to double check on a couple of words. How do you spell "ricocheted" and "hemorrhaging" anyhow?

Writing, the simple act of putting down on paper what you know, what you think. and what you dream is a rewarding experience. The magic of words doesn't depend upon public exposure. The satisfaction derived from creating sentences that sing is at least equal to that one gains from arranging musical notes. And putting together paragraphs and pages that combine to express a new idea is as thrilling as driving a golf ball 200 yards off the tee.

— Leonard K. Knott
Writing for the Joy of It
(Writer's Digest Books, 1983),
p. 18

And we are writing this that our joy
may be complete.
— 1 John 1:4

Any plans for writing something you've been thinking about for a long time? Like an essay, a poem, letters, family history, a cookbook, a bedtime story, an article, something in your journal . . . or anything else at all. Why not begin this very day?

FIXED, SURE, AND REGULAR

Changing planes and airlines at Minneapolis, we are notified that our eight-passenger Cessna has a flat tire. My arrival at Moline will be delayed. Rats!

So we switched to Mississippi Valley Airlines (Shades of Bob Newhart!) Flying along at what seems like "tree-top" level, I can see some great running spots. There's a nifty area! A quiet road along that meandering Wisconsin River.

My daily vacation (run) this morning was so routine I guess I should have suspected some snafus the rest of the day. It's great to do something each day that is "fixed, sure and regular," because it doesn't depend on anyone else. Just me. Puts a little more order in my life.

Running . . . brings not just physical benefits but a number of psychological benefits. It does not bring either, however, unless it is done regularly. From the beginning, therefore, make running a habit. Set aside a time solely for running, and make it long enough to give yourself plenty of time for dressing, warming up, running, cooling down, taking a leisurely shower and dressing again. Running is more fun if you don't have to rush through it.

> — James F. Fixx *The Complete Book of Running* (Random House, 1977), p. 71

> Jesus Christ is the same yesterday and today and for ever.
> — Hebrews 13:8

What do you do for your daily vacation?

LET ME BE WHAT I CAN BE

Later today I'll be bringing the invocation at the opening ceremonies for the Fargo Regional Special Olympics. I want to feel the atmosphere of the area, so this morning's run finds me circling the New Field House at North Dakota State University where the festivities will take place.

One hundred and sixty young women and men will recite the Special Olympic Oath after I say my words. Mayor Lindgren will lead us. It goes like this:

Let me be what I can be,
Let me do what I can do.

I'm grateful to the Kennedy family for developing the Special Olympics. I don't know how anyone can participate in these events and not feel deeply moved. I like the idea of having official "huggers," volunteers who hug each person when they have finished their race or swim. That way everyone wins.

My friend, Chaplain Dave Hurtt, helped with some of the wording for my prayer, and my run today helps my thoughts click into their final order. Here's what I'll be saying:

O Creator of the Universe
 . . . and of us all.
Thank you for the joy of this day.
For the fun of . . .
  — Running fast and jumping high.
  — Swimming wet and throwing long.
  — Doing our best . . . giving it our all.

We are happy for this chance to show our stuff!

Just to be here is a blessing.
  Just to be alive is holy.

We are thankful for the support and care we enjoy as our community comes together to celebrate life.

Grant us help to be happy with whatever we do . . . and that just to be here is to win.

Thanks. Oh, Thanks! For all these friends. Amen

> Then the eyes of the blind
>> shall be opened,
> and the ears of the deaf unstopped;
> then shall the lame . . . leap like
>> a hart . . .
>> — Isaiah 35:5-6

Why not reach out this week and become friends with someone who is developmentally or physically disabled?

COMPULSION

My compulsion puts me on the road again this morning, even though spring has been set back by an untimely return of Old Man Winter. You might say today has "summer skies with winter's eyes."

And yesterday was one of those days when I overscheduled myself. I'm tired. Think I'll just run about twenty minutes today. Build up my reserve of strength to run longer tomorrow. I've been around long enough to know that some days are going to be like this. No use trying to explain them. I guess I've learned to just accept such times. If my "inner monitor" didn't make me feel guilty, I'd probably still be in bed.

Normally, when I receive many letters I complain that I am too busy, and when I receive none I complain about lack of attention; when I work a lot I complain about lack of time to study and pray, when I work little I feel guilty for not making a contribution . . . But during the past few weeks I have felt an inner distance which has allowed me to see my compulsions and therefore to lose them, and I have experienced some new inner freedom.

> — Henri J. M. Nouwen
> *The Genesee Diary*
> (Image Books, 1981), p. 202

Go to the ant, O sluggard;
consider her ways, and be wise.

How long will you lie, there, O
sluggard?
When will you arise from your sleep?
— Proverbs 6:6, 9

What is one of your compulsions? How do you deal with it?

YOU DON'T HAVE TO SIT ON THAT BENCH

Ten minutes from our hotel, my run brings me to Hennepin Avenue and Harmon Place. Loring Park is beautiful this morning. There are many benches everywhere and a bridge right in the middle I want to run across. As I do I meet a biker.

The power of last night's play at the Guthrie is yet with me. That final scene of "Master Harold . . . and the Boys," will not leave my mind's lens. I can still hear Sam (played by James Earl Jones) speaking about a "whites only" spot, to young Hally, say, "You don't have to sit on that bench. You can get up, stand up, walk away from it any time you choose."

The ambiguity and ambivalence of life, and its clarity and simple joy, are contrasted well for me by last night's theatre and this morning's drama.

> The truth is that our civilization is not Christian; it is a tragic compound of great ideal and fearful practice, of high assurance and desperate anxiety, of loving charity and fearful clutching of possessions.
> — Alan Paton
> Cry, the Beloved Country

> I do not understand my own actions.
> For I do not do what I want, but I do
> the very thing I hate.
> — Romans 7:15

Do you think the worlds of "people of color" and of whites will be bridged in your lifetime? Why do you think that?

IN BETWEEN FUNERALS

Last night we gathered at the Hanson-Runsvold Funeral Home and I led a memorial service for Selma Brothers, age ninety-four. Later this morning I'll be conducting the funeral for my old friend, Clara Maser, age ninety. So, as I run today, it is in between funerals, so to speak. Causes a guy to think a little. On the roads is where my mind is as clear as it ever is. When I'm sailing along I know that I am body and soul, and that my forty-five minutes of daily adventure gives me a glimpse of eternity.

I used Alfred Lord Tennyson's masterpiece, "Crossing the Bar" last night at Selma's service, and probably will use it again today, at Clara's. It speaks to me these days with a special force.

Sunset and evening star,
    And one clear call for me!
And may there be no moaning of the bar,
    When I put out to sea.

But such a tide as moving seems asleep,
    Too full for sound and foam,
When that which drew from out the boundless deep
    Turns again home.

Twilight and evening bell,
    And after that the dark!
And may there be no sadness of farewell,
    When I embark;

For though from out our bourne of Time and Place
    The flood may bear me far,
I hope to see my Pilot face to face
    When I have crost the bar.

— Alfred, Lord Tennyson (1889)

For a thousand years in thy sight
    are but as yesterday when it is
        past,
  or as a watch in the night.
— Psalm 90:4

What is one of your favorite passages of Scripture or other pieces of literature which give you a glimpse of the reality of eternity?

CHURCH CHOIRS

Who has more fun than church choirs? Ron told me that when Dave was in training for the run around Lake Mille Lacs, he would often run in from his home quite a way down the road. One night he was late and one of the choir members suggested, "Maybe he hit a deer." I love it. I love it. Only in Northern Minnesota!

Then yesterday, I was speaking at Colfax and during refreshment time heard someone say that their choir was meeting at 9:00 p.m. since most of the farm folk were in the fields as long as possible, "making hay while the sun shines." As a gentle protest, one of the members of that singing group, a teacher in town, showed up in his pajamas. I love that too! My hat is off to that lover of life.

Over my years as a pastor associated with choirs, I realize that most have been support groups every bit as much as singing groups. How fine! Who, indeed, does have more fun than church choirs?

Overheard at a church music conference:
"If God gave you a good voice, why not show your gratitude by singing in your church choir? And if you didn't receive a good voice, join the choir as a way of getting even!"

Praise the Lord!
Sing to the Lord a new song,
    his praise in the assembly of the
        faithful.
                                    — Psalm 149:1

What is one memory you have of a church choir you have been in or known?

NAMES

I'm buzzing along on North Dakota 32, on my way to speak to the Ransom County Homemaker's gathering at Lisbon. And I'm thinking how great it would be to be running on such a lonesome road. I enjoy "bombing around" North Dakota in my little blue Fiat, but I'd rather be running.

Suddenly a sign catches my eye:

Buttzville 3

Wouldn't Johnny Carson have fun with this name!?

BUECHNER
It is my name. It is pronounced Beekner. If somebody mispronounces it in some foolish way, I have the feeling that what's foolish is me. If somebody forgets it, I feel that it's I who am forgotten. There's something about it that embarrasses me. I can't imagine myself with any other name — Held, say, or Merrill, or Hlavacek. If my name were different, I would be different. When I tell somebody my name, I have given him a hold over me that he didn't have before. If he calls it out, I stop, look, and listen whether I want to or not.

In the Book of Exodus, God tells Moses that his name is Yahweh, and God hasn't had a peaceful moment since.
> — Frederick Buechner
> *Wishful Thinking*
> (Harper and Row, 1973), p. 12

> Then Moses said to God, "If I come to the people of Israel and say to them, 'The God of your fathers has sent me to you,' and they ask me, 'What is his name?' what shall I say to them?"
> — Exodus 3:13

If you could take a different name, what would it be?

THE IMPORTANCE OF FRIENDS

Seeing my friend, Tom, this morning reminds me that "Friends are forever." How great! How fine! How nourishing for our existence.

I see him from about a block away as he heads for South High. It is 6:00 a.m. No doubt his swim team has an early practice. I believe he's coached for over thirty years. As we close the gap between us, I am thinking how good it is to see him. It's been over a year I think. There is a warmth as we stop a moment and greet each other. Like it was just yesterday, we had talked.

I keep reading about research coming out of the California Department of Mental Health which declares that friends and other supportive relationships are as important to our *physical* well-being as they are to our emotional health.

With that thought in mind, here are two ideas that have worked their way into my life style:

> *According to new medical research, excessive stress in our lives is at the root of fifty to eighty percent of all illness. If we can find ways to reduce the stress in our lives, we cannot only help cut down . . . medical costs, but we can actually prevent many illnesses from occurring in the first place. Friends are an important factor in modifying the negative effects of excessive stress in our lives.*

> — From a brochure called "Friends Can Be Good Medicine" California Department of Mental Health, 1981

"Payments to experts are made in dollars, but more agonizingly, perhaps, in self-esteem."

> — Mary C. Howell
> *Helping Ourselves: Families and the Human Network*
> (Beacon Press, 1975), p. 71

> Peace be to you. The friends greet you. Greet the friends, every one of them.

> — 3 John 15

Who would you consider to be your "best friend" today?

SEX IS A HOT ITEM

There are lots of things I encounter as I run the streets of Fargo — Moorhead. Golf balls, keys, coins, a pair of perfectly good pliers, and lots more. Today I see again a "Girlie" magazine. These show up quite often on the roads. I'm guessing it's because they get tossed before someone gets home. This one is almost "brand new" so I can scan it easier than some others.

I think of the "flap" about the sexuality programs at LSS of Minnesota this spring, and I recall the time Judge Davies spoke at our Ministerial Association Meeting, sharing some pornographic films and magazines. Largest attendance we *ever* had!

Sex is a hot item.

Few would doubt that this is a time of transition in our understanding of human sexuality. The confusion about sexual morals and mores is the more obvious evidence of this. But there is something else. For too long the bulk of Christian reflection about sexuality has asked an essentially one-directional question: what does Christian faith have to say about our lives as sexual beings? Now we are beginning to realize that the enterprise must be a genuinely two-directional affair. The first question is essential, and we must continue unfailingly to press it. But at the same time it must be joined by, indeed interwoven with, a companion query: what does our experience as sexual human beings mean for the way in which we understand and attempt to live out the faith? What does it mean that we as body-selves are invited to participate in the reality of God?

> — James B. Nelson
> *Embodiment*
> (Augsburg, 1978), pp. 8-9

Behold, you are beautiful, my love,
behold, you are beautiful!
-- Song of Solomon 4:1

What is the most helpful book you have encountered on human sexuality? If you haven't read it, try Jim Nelson's *Embodiment*. Its subtitle is: *An Approach to Sexuality and Christian Theology.* I recommend it highly.

(Another is *The Human Face of God* by John A. T. Robinson. Very helpful also.)

CURING OURSELVES

It's icy this morning and the footing is treacherous on University Drive. I need to run very slowly. Part of me says I ought to take a day off and not risk injury. But I now assume that's my "shadow side" speaking. I really do need to run every day. My addiction is calling.

A middle-aged client was complaining of his daily fatigue. His work exhausted him, and every day when he returned home he was fragmented. "The only thing which helps me," he said, "is when I climb up the mountain right near my house." It was a modest mountain, really just a large hill, which he could hike up and back in about an hour. "Then why don't you climb it every day?" I asked. "Every day?" he replied in astonishment. "Why, I thought that would be a cop-out, using something as a crutch." I answered, "Every day you become a little bit ill, and every day you need to cure yourself. If this is the way you cure yourself, then do it." My friend now climbs his mountain five times a week, rain or shine, and each time returns renewed. One could say he cures himself of his psychic ills by using his body. It is a small example of the healing potential that lies in the proper relationship with our physical self.
— John A. Sanford
Healing and Wholeness
(Paulist Press, 1977), p. 127

And David danced before the Lord
with all his might . . . "
— 2 Samuel 6:14

What is your favorite physical activity which helps clear the cobwebs from your mind?

BE A FRIEND TO YOURSELF

I'm on my way to Westhope and Minot for some meetings, so I'm running at Lakota this morning. There's a friendly east wind blowing. Today's five helps me sort out yesterday's meeting. I spoke to the Counseling Department at NDSU and saw there a wall poster that was a "double image" picture of Garfield, the now famous cat. Underneath it said, "Be a Friend to Yourself."

I shared with them a phenomenon I have recently firmed up in my mind. That is, in order to be a source of nourishment for another (a friend), we first have to be a friend to ourselves. And in order to affect a change in another we need to first make some changes in ourselves. When we do that, an atmosphere or aura of possibility of change surrounds the other one and makes it easier for them to alter their behavior. I also said that Carl Rogers' life-changing concept of "unconditional positive regard" ought to beam inward to ourselves, as well as outward toward others.

> One fundamental thing, for example, is to meet your own expectations. If you have housework or homework to do, and you are tempted to let it slide, ask yourself how you will feel if you put it off. If you sense that you will be a little disgusted with yourself, then go ahead and do the job, and let yourself savor the feeling you get from having done it. Enjoy the experience of being in charge of yourself.
>
> — Mildred Newman and Bernard
> Berkowitz, How to Be
> Your Own Best Friend
> (Ballantine, 1971), p. 32

> "You shall love the Lord your God
> with all your heart, and with all your
> soul, and with all your strength, and
> with all your mind; and your neighbor
> as yourself."
>
> — St. Luke 10:26

Have you been a "friend to yourself" lately? Talk about one way you have . . . or haven't.

A MINOR REBIRTH

I know I'll be asked again soon. "Why *do* you run anyway?" It happens at least once a week it seems. But next time I'll be ready. Reading one of John Sanford's nourishing books I came across this great answer I can give. He says just what I intend:

> *Jogging and long-distance running are two other forms of exercise that can have a rhythm. The goal here is to achieve a constant flow of energy and feel the rhythm of one's body, and experience the deep, even breathing that comes from such forms of movement. Under these conditions the entire psyche enters into an unusual state. The long-distance runner frequently reports discernible states of consciousness. At first there may be the feeling of effort, then sometimes a brief period of depression, followed by a strange euphoria, and then an unusual state of inner equilibrium is achieved in which all sorts of thoughts flow spontaneously through consciousness. At the same time that the heart pumps blood through the veins and arteries, and energy moves through the body, psychic energy also moves from the unconscious through consciousness and back again. When the total experience ends with a renewing shower, the effect can be like a minor rebirth.*
> — John A. Sanford
> *Healing and Wholeness*
> (Paulist Press, 1977),
> pp. 130-131

> And in the morning, a great while
> before day, he rose and went out to
> a lonely place, and there he prayed.
> — St. Mark 1:35

What activity do you have to do that gives you a feeling or euphoria sometimes?

FREE SPACE

It's just after my run this morning and I feel like reading a little Henri Nouwen. A while back he spent seven months participating fully in the daily life and routine at the Abbey of the Genesee in Upstate New York. That included work and prayer. Out of that experience he was able to discover, as he says, "a quiet stream underneath the fluctuating affirmations and rejections of my little world."

As I pick up and begin reading where I left off, from his daily diary of that experience, I come across these words. As a pastor, and at the stage of life I'm in, they speak to me strongly. He is reflecting on the life of Thomas Merton:

> *He indeed made his own life available to others to help them find their own — and not his — way. In this sense, he was and still is a true minister, creating the free space where others can enter and discover God's voice in their lives.*
> — Henri J. M. Nouwen
> *The Genesee Diary*
> (Image Books/Doubleday,
> 1981), p. 184

> ". . . You will know the truth, and the
> truth will make you free."
> — St. John 8:32

What is a concept that has helped make some "free space" in your life? Who is a person who has done that?

THE POET AND THE RUNNER

Robert Frost and Bill Rodgers. Poetry and "Poetry-in-Motion."
How great! How fine! To be able to run close to these two men! Our
vacation has taken us here. Today I'm running along part of the Boston
Marathon route on Commonwealth Avenue. A good feeling. I visited
Bill Rodgers' Running Center, too. Now I can say, "Yes, I've run in
Boston."

And just a few days ago we stumbled across Robert Frost's home
in Franconia, New Hampshire. Shirley and I were the only ones there!
What a pleasant "plus" to our already fantastic fall vacation.

To run in Boston and Franconia where these two disparate men
(both important in my life) made and are making tracks, leaves me
awed . . . and thankful for life.

The woods are lovely, dark, and deep,
But I have promises to keep,
And miles to go before I sleep,
And miles to go before I sleep.

— Robert Frost, the closing lines of:
"Stopping by Woods on a
Snowy Evening."
The Poetry of Robert Frost
(Holt, Rinehart and Winston,
1969), pp. 224-225

(Bill Rodgers) is . . . five feet eight and a half inches tall
and weighs 125 pounds, exactly what he weighed in junior
high school. His hair is sandy blond, his teeth are small and
startlingly regular. As he runs, he suggests an extraordinary
mechanical harmony, every part working in diligent concert
with every other. His arms rock like pendulums. His feet strike
the ground softly, at the heel, then roll forward until only a
spot of toe links his body to the earth. Then he floats through
the air for an unbelievably long time until another heel finally
sinks gently to the pavement. As he moves, his head neither
rises nor falls but acts as if it were gyroscopically stabilized.

"If I ever stopped running I'd feel terrible," he says, "as
if I were slowly decomposing. I enjoy being fit. There's a feel-
ing of independence about it. If I get a flat tire and am ten miles

from a gas station I can just run there, instead of sitting for three hours and freezing."

> — James F. Fixx
> *The Complete Book of Running* (Random House, 1977), p. 218

Therefore, since we are surrounded by so great a cloud of witnesses, let us also lay aside every weight, and sin which clings so closely, and let us run with perseverance the race that is set before us.

> — Hebrews 12:1

Name a couple of people you would like to meet.

AFTER SUICIDE

I'm feeling alive and in touch with myself and creation after an invigorating and adventurous forty-minute run this morning. It is five below zero with a thirty-mile-per-hour wind. That puts the wind-chill factor at somewhere between forty-five and sixty below! There's about fifteen inches of snow on the ground — and still coming down. A regular North Dakota blizzard.

All this encounter with the elements is lost, however, as I step into the kitchen from the back porch. "Pick up the phone, Roger!" Shirley is calling to me from the bedroom. I can tell by her tone that it's something dreadful. "Brad has committed suicide, and your Dad's on the line."

O God, be with Marge and Neb and the rest of the family!

A member of your immediate family or the larger family of those dear to you has purposely ended his of her life. Your loved one has been permanently torn away, leaving a gaping wound in your life tht you may doubt will ever heal. Now you are left behind to undergo the agony of acute bereavement, a grief punctuated by spasms of guilt, anger, bewilderment, and shame. Suicide, that whispered taboo which only happens to other families, has happened to yours . . .

It's too late to stop the suicide that has scarred your life. The time for "prevention" or "intervention" has passed. However, the time is right to begin your crucial process of "postvention" — that process after a suicide during which your family works toward emotional recovery and readjustment to healthy living. The suicidal death of your family member forces you to ask different questions, express unusual emotions, and face difficult fears. That's why "postvention" is for you.
— John H. Hewett
After Suicide
(Westminster, 1980), p. 11

"I am the resurrection and the life."
— St. John 11:25

Recall someone you know who took their own life. Remember the family in prayer.

CATS ARE ALWAYS ON THE WRONG SIDE OF DOORS

I have just finished a slow, gentle, mind-clearing run, and in an hour or so I'll be leaving to speak to the folks at Ottawa Church near Aneta, North Dakota. Judy Rusten, who has been coordinating the event, sent me a note last week that makes me nostalgic about the parish ministry. "Go west of Sharon," she writes, "about six miles and when the road turns south go straight west on the gravel road for four miles. The church is right along the gravel road." Our first parish in Hines, Minnesota, was along a gravel road, too.

While I was still a parish pastor, I thought it would be good to be with Lutheran Social Services. Now that I'm with LSS I miss the parish. My feelings remind me of something I read the other day: "Cats are always," the article said, "on the wrong side of doors." How true! How true! And right now that seems to describe me too. I wonder if other folks identify with that trait of our feline friends. I bet so.

On quiet afternoons, I like to watch the white cat sit still as a ceramic vase, ears swiveling like radar dishes to catch the sounds of birds and animals inaudible to me. Then he stands up, arches briefly, and looks at the door. He can work the latch himself, but why bother? "Meow?" he asks. Cats are always on the wrong side of doors. He pauses while I hold the door, testing the wind, never hurrying. Then he trots off, tail high, and never looking back.

— Kathleen Kilgore
"The Incredible World of Cats"
Yankee, October 1980, p. 151

Be content with what you have.
— Hebrews 13:5

Can you think of a wise old saying that says about the same thing as "Cats are always on the wrong side of doors?"

DON'T JUDGE A RUNNER'S HAPPINESS BY THE WIDTH OF THE GRIN

"You never see a happy runner." "Have you ever seen a runner with a smile on his face?" How many times have we heard similar phrases? It happened again just yesterday. It seems like it's almost always a sort of "chubby" person who says these things. I never knew before quite how to counter. But a welcome letter from an old friend today helped clarify my thoughts on this. He had just completed a tough marathon.

"You never see a happy runner," a camping friend had told me and I took strong exception. How do you measure happiness anyway? I was extremely tired, my left foot was sore, left ankle ached some, both hips were aching — no smile on my face, just dried tears. As soon as I'd stopped running my calf muscles cramped up and I had trouble breathing. However . . . I had won the battle against the course, taken seven minutes off my previous best marathon time, and at age fifty-nine qualified to run with the elite at Boston. For years I'll be able to look at my plaque, or finishing photo, or just mentally re-live the struggle, and be happy . . . Don't judge a runner's happiness by the width of the grin.
— Wilson St. Martin, Murray, Utah
(Personal correspondence)

Nat King Cole used to sing a beautiful song called "Laughing on the outside, crying on the inside." Maybe for most of us runners, we could change that and sing, "Crying on the outside, rejoicing on the inside." Wil certainly could.

. . . Let us run with perseverance the race that is set before us.
— Hebrews 12:1

Can you think of another situation, besides running, when facial expression does not reveal inner feelings?

DON'T SWEAT THE SMALL STUFF

Woodbury, Connecticut. On vacation. The older woman in Room No. 4, right next to us in The Curtis House, has gotten up at 6 a.m. both days. She plays solitaire, works on a jig-saw puzzle, watches TV . . . and all the guests go by her room. I bet she's a regular resident here. Maybe the owner, or the owner's wife or mother. She smiles and nods each time I go by. Her contented look and relaxed schedule say to me, "Here is one who learned to live with a minimum of stress."

I do like this place. We have a spacious room, a good writing desk and a great dining area. The Innkeeper tells us it was built before 1754!

Three Rules for Dealing With Stress:

1. *Don't sweat the small stuff.*
2. *It's all small stuff.*
3. *If you can't fight and you can't flee, flow.*
   — Dr. Robert Eliot
   University of Nebraska

". . . Do not be anxious about your
life . . ."
   — Matthew 6:25

What is something you like to do that helps you relax and unwind?

WE BURIED MOM TODAY

Grandview Cemetery. Aptly named. High on a hilltop, just outside Fayette, Iowa. January 26, 1984. Thirty-one degrees. A gentle winter day. The snow-filled arms of the evergreens surround us as we pay a final tribute to our Mom. Marge, Jer, Neb, and I take turns reading, . . . "In sure and certain hope of the resurrection to eternal life . . . we commend to almighty God our mother, Elsie . . . earth to earth, ashes to ashes . . . " She was born and grew up only a mile from here, and there is a comfort to this place and to this day. Elsie Mae Fussell Prescott has finally stepped beyond the boundaries of her life, and her troubles are gone now. She has come to the true ease of herself. So long, Mom. We love you. We'll miss you. May your memory be blessed forever.

When Marge called to tell me Mom had died, I went to my study and put these thoughts together for the day's *Warmline* message:

A new white quilt covers the ground this morning. I admire its downy beauty from the kitchen window. I see several sparrows huddled in our backyard bushes . . . their feathers all fluffed up like shivering men huddled in overcoats. Putting on my overshoes I go outside and fill up the holder with seeds and grain, and spill some for extra measure. Soon the yard and trees are alive with sound; a chattering convention of sparrows, nuthatches, and one I can't identify. I have seen their need and responded.

This morning, I am also the bird in the bush, the one with needs. I am sad and feeling alone, and wondering who will see my need and respond. I recall that Jesus told his disciples he would send them a Comforter (John 14:16) and that he would neither leave them nor forsake them. (Hebrews 13:5) You and I have these promises when life grows desperate, and we feel overwhelmed. Our heavenly Creator knows our needs and will supply them. We can trust that process.

And now Shirley's arms surround me.

— Roger Prescott

Look at the birds of the air: they
neither sow nor reap nor gather into
barns, and yet your heavenly Father

feeds them. Are you not of more
value than they?

— Matthew 7:26

Recall and describe a cemetery that has meaning for you.

FAMILY MEMORIES

For the past few days I've noticed our neighbors are in various stages of completion in getting their winter "storm windows" on. I haven't even started. I'm running so well these days I'd rather spend time on the roads. But I'll get to it. It's going on the "list" next week. "Begin storm windows!"

In the meantime, seeing all this window activity around has incited my mind to leapfrog back a few years to something Ruthie once said.

I've never been known as a "fixer." In fact, when anything breaks, if I can't fix it with a little glue or a reinforcing nail, it will stay unfixed for a long time. When the upstairs window in Ruth's room broke I fashioned a replacement by buying a simple pane of glass and attaching it permanently to the sash. No matter that it couldn't go up and down. Another window in the room could. That ought to be enough.

We were eating supper one night and the talk turned to when I was going to finish getting the storm windows on. "It's getting cold in my room, Dad," said Dave. Then Ruth said, "And you know that pane of glass in my room that serves as a window . . . " She never got the rest of the sentence out. Suzy began laughing. "That pane of glass that serves as a window?" "Ha, ha, ha, ha, ha." We all began laughing then, when we realized the subtlety of what was being said. Another one of Dad's makeshift-Jerry-built-Rube Goldberg type repairs became famous.

When we get together as a family we still can get a good laugh just by mentioning, "You know that pane of glass that serves as a window . . ." Such fun. Such good memories.

(As I write this — May 1984 — that "pane of glass" still serves.)

— Roger Prescott

And the windows of the heavens
were opened.
— Genesis 7:11

Do you recall any unique windows in your life? Tell about one.

SPEED WORK

People tell me I'm a slow runner. I know that. I know that. But I like to be slow. Every time I get the bug and try some speed work, something happens. A cold. A problem at the office. I guess I just like the comfortable rhythm I've been in for several years. Some may call it a "rut." Not me. It's more like "consistent." My racing time for the 10 K is about the same as one of my training runs. Nine minutes a mile.

The other day, though, I heard one of my kids talking about me to a friend. "My Dad likes to pace himself. He starts out slowly, and then tapers off." Ouch! I've just got to begin a little speed work.

Mike Laws' friends are still trying to convince him to con-sider some speedwork, but he is sticking to the daily ten-mile runs he prefers and seems unconcerned about his times:

"If I never ran another race, I'd still run every day, because I like the way it makes me feel. I started running because I wanted to improve the way I looked, but it's done much more for my insides than my outside. If I just want to clear my head I can go out to enjoy the woods, the beaches, the scenic places. If I need to concentrate, I can zero in on a problem and solve it before my run's over. What I'm completely incapable of doing when I run is carrying along my worries, which have never done me any good anyway."

> — Mike Law, Restauranteur, as
> quoted in "Road to Success" by
> C. Edward Houser,
> *Runner's World Magazine*,
> August 1980, p. 124

". . . the race is not to the swift . . ."
> — Ecclesiastes 9:11

The world record for the mile is three minutes and forty-seven seconds, set by Sebastian Coe on the twenty-eighth of August 1981. How long do you think it would take you to run a mile?

CARS WE HAVE KNOWN

Our family has had some strange cars in our time. Today as I trek down Eddy Court I hear a vehicle coming up on me that sounds like a truck. When it passes I see that it is an old clunk of a Chevy without a muffler or a left-front fender. My thoughts skip back to some of *our* "bombs."

The "Green Giant" *(1963 Chrysler)*
Famous for its huge size and errant windshield washers. They shot the water right over the roof onto the rear window!

The "White Knight" *(1961 Ford)*
Known for the magic method of opening the window on the driver's side. Slam the door and it would drop deftly to the bottom of the door frame. Flashy! And this auto shook embarrassingly when it idled!

'74 Valiant
It had been clobbered so many times that the roof was the only part that had not been replaced. Most of the kids learned to drive in this one. In its last days it moved sort of sideways down the road.

'60 Chev
This car ran so well the floorboards wore out before the engine. When we'd drive through a puddle, water hitting the exhaust pipe would put steam all through the interior. A regular sauna! Shirley took her Utah driver's test in this one and had to pull the clutch out by hand. She passed. The inspector must have thought if anyone could drive this clunk, she could drive anything.

"The Rambler"
Nothing worked right on this one. We only had it for a short time after the steering wheel came off putting us in the ditch. That was shortly after the drive shaft fell out one day right on Beacon Hill Road.

'49 Ford Pick-up

Used by David for getting around in Fargo. Hauled a lot of junk to the dump and will always be remembered with love as it was "Dave's First Car." It died one day in a cloud of blue smoke on Highway 10, returning from Detroit Lakes.

> The chariots rage in the streets,
> they rush to and fro through the
> squares.
>   — Nahum 2:4

Describe an idiosyncrasy of one of the cars you have owned.